bodyworks

Published in 2007 by Murdoch Books Pty Limited
www.murdochbooks.com.au

Murdoch Books Australia
Pier 8/9
23 Hickson Road
Millers Point NSW 2000
Phone: +61 (0) 2 8220 2000
Fax: +61 (0) 2 8220 2558

Murdoch Books UK Limited
Erico House
6th Floor North
93–99 Upper Richmond Road
Putney, London SW15 2TG
Phone: +44 (0) 20 8785 5995
Fax: +44 (0) 20 8785 5985

Chief Executive: Juliet Rogers
Publishing Director: Kay Scarlett

Commissioning Editor: Diana Hill
Art direction and design concept: Vivien Valk
Design: Michelle Cutler
Project Manager and Editor: Rhiain Hull
Production: Maiya Levitch
Recipes: Nerys Purchon pages 22, 24–5, 27, 28–30, 36, 38–9, 41 (top), 42, 49–52, 55, 57 (top), 58, 65–6, 68, 81–2, 84, 90–2, 95, 96 (bottom), 98 (top), 102, 107, 110, 118, 120–1, 123–6, 128–9, 131–4, 138, 140, 142–3, 145, 148 (top), 150–1, 154, 160–1, 164, 167–8, 170 (top), 172–3 and 175 (top); Cheryl Ross pages 32–3, 35, 41 (bottom), 43, 44, 46–7, 57 (bottom), 59–60, 62–3, 67, 70–1, 73–6, 78–9, 83, 86–7, 89, 96 (top), 97, 98 (bottom), 104–5, 108–9, 112–113, 115–17, 139, 146–7, 148 (bottom), 153, 155–6, 162, 165, 169, 170 (bottom), 175 (bottom), 178–180, 182–3, 186–8.
Photographers: Alan Benson back cover and pages 4, 6, 8, 18, 20, 23, 26, 31, 37, 40, 48, 53, 56, 64, 80, 85, 93, 94, 103, 114, 119, 122, 127, 141, 144, 149, 152, 158, 166 and 189; Greg Delves pages 103, 174, 130 and 135; Natasha Milne front cover and pages 9, 21, 34, 45, 61, 69, 72, 77, 88, 99, 100–1, 106, 111, 137, 157, 159, 163, 171, 176–7, 181, 184–5.
Stylists: Justine Brown back cover and pages 4, 6, 8, 18, 20, 23, 26, 31, 37, 40, 48, 53, 56, 64, 80, 85, 93, 94, 114, 119, 122, 127, 141, 144, 149, 152, 158, 166, 189; Jane Campsie pages 103, 130, 135, 174; Sarah O'Brien front cover and pages 9, 21, 34, 45, 61, 69, 72, 77, 88, 99, 100–1, 106, 111, 137, 157, 159, 163, 171, 176–7, 181, 184–5.

National Library of Australia Cataloguing-in-Publication Data
Bodyworks. Includes index.
ISBN 978 1 74045 823 8. ISBN 1 74045 823 0.
1. Skin - Care and hygiene. 2. Beauty, Personal. 3. Herbal cosmetics. I. Hull, Rhiain. 646.726

Printed by Midas Printing (Asia) Ltd. in 2007. PRINTED IN CHINA.

IMPORTANT: Some of the recipes in this book contain borax, a natural powdered mineral salt. Recipes containing borax should not be used for infants and children, pregnant women or those with sensitive skin.

bodyworks

restoring wellbeing with homemade
organic lotions, potions and balms

MURDOCH BOOKS

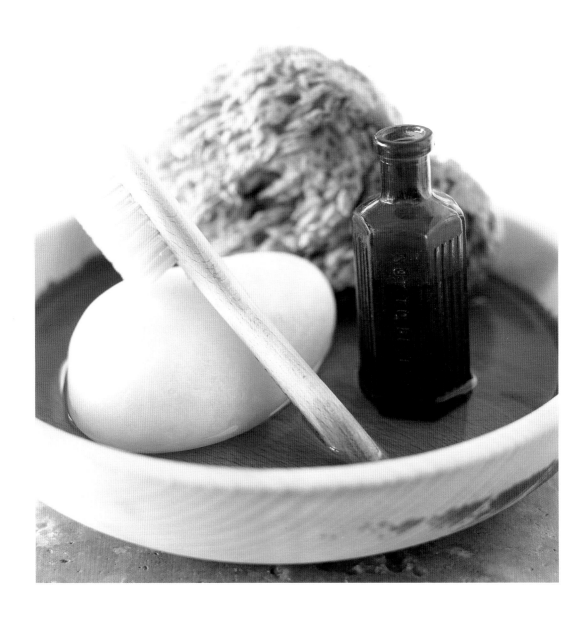

contents

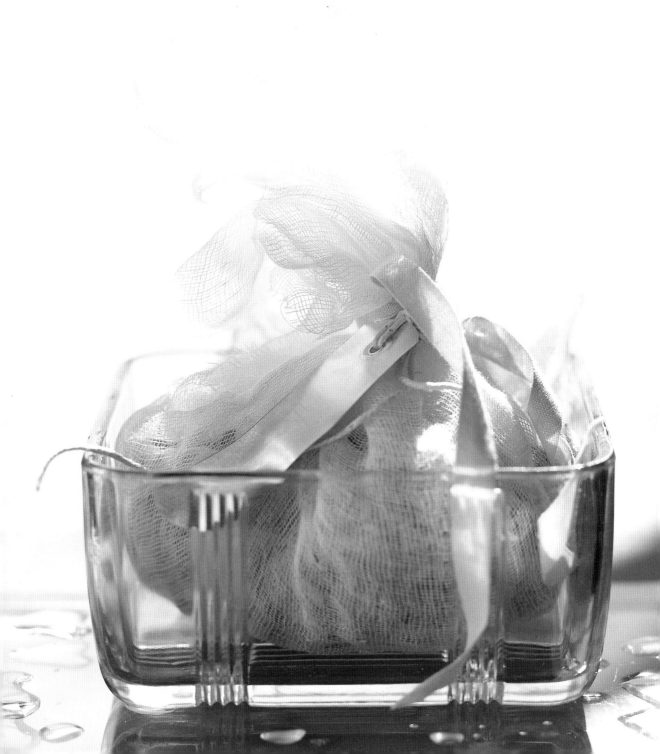

introduction

There are many benefits in making your own body care products. Beauty preparations made from natural ingredients can give us everything we need to nourish and pamper our skin.

Many chemicals are used in commercial skincare and hair care products, which do not contain any beneficial nutrients and may irritate the skin. Nature provides us with all the essential vitamins and minerals to promote healthy, glowing skin and shiny hair.

Feeding your skin is just as important as feeding your body. All the recipes in this book are formulated to deliver anti-oxidants, vitamins, minerals and enzymes to hydrate, nourish and protect your skin and hair against cellular damage. The treatments can have a lasting revitalizing effect if you use them regularly.

Using herbs, vegetables, fruit and other natural produce to create your own body care products can be exciting, rewarding and can bring you great joy.

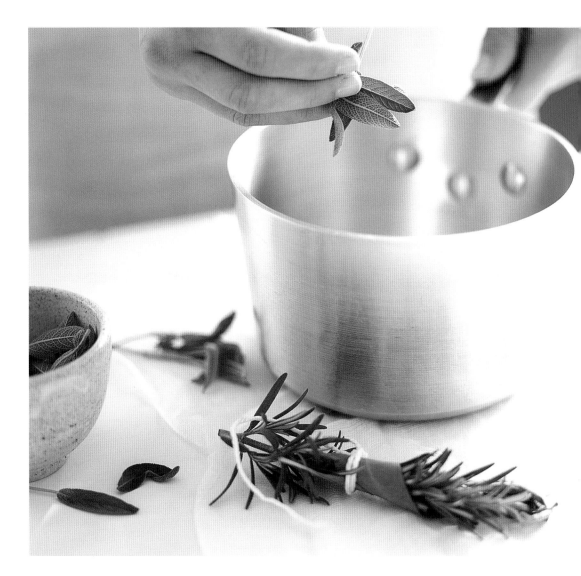

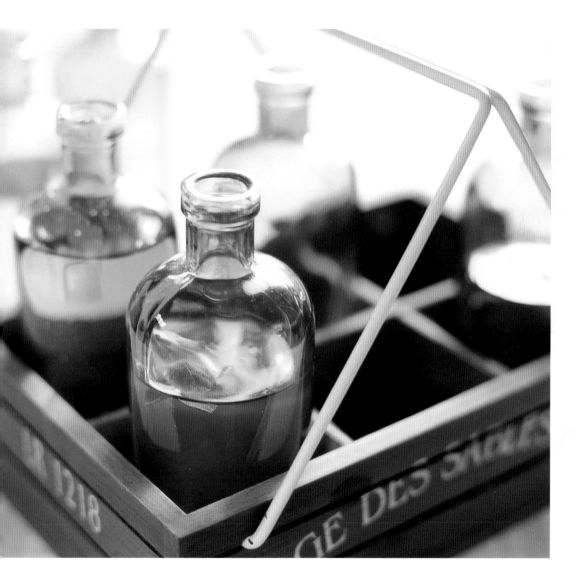

the basics

what should you put on your skin?

A list of ingredients and a few of their properties is provided below to help you when creating your own recipes. All these wonderful natural ingredients can be found in your kitchen cupboard, garden, or health food stores.

HERBAL TEAS

chamomile tea   Soothing, calming. Good for sensitive skin.

parsley tea   Great for congested skin. A good skin lightener.

raspberry tea   Whitens the skin. Good for brown spots. Can be used as a toner.

HERBS

Many different herbs such as comfrey★ (healing, anti-inflammatory) and chamomile (calming, hydrating and soothing) have great properties for skincare.

calendula   Contains salicylic acid, carotenoids and phytosterols. Anti-inflammatory. Calendula-infused oil is very helpful for acne, eczema, wounds, dry or cracked skin and varicose veins.

ginkgo biloba   Anti-oxidant and skin hydrator. It regulates the sebaceous glands, which provide natural lubrication for the skin and hair.

ginseng   Anti-oxidant. Anti-inflammatory properties. Firms the skin.

* Comfrey is a restricted substance in some countries.

| witch hazel | An astringent. Softening. Balances the oil sebum of the skin. Anti-inflammatory and anti-couperose (decreases redness in the face). Readily available in liquid form from pharmacies. |

SOLID FATS AND WAXES

| beeswax | An emulsifier. Contains anti-allergic and anti-inflammatory properties. |

| cocoa butter | Nourishes, softens and conditions the skin. Great in moisturizers. |

| shea butter | Very nourishing and penetrating. Excellent for extremely dry skin. Good for psoriasis and eczema. |

ANTI-OXIDANTS

| green tea | A powerful anti-oxidant that helps to reduce swelling. Calms sensitive skin. |

| vitamin E | An important anti-oxidant that contains tocopherol acetate. Helps protect skin cells. Makes a good preservative for creams (as little as 0.5% can be used). Very moisturizing and great in soothing and healing masks. Is readily available in liquid form. |

VEGETABLE OILS

| apricot kernel oil | Contains minerals and vitamins. Good source of vitamin A. |

avocado oil	Contains vitamins, protein, lecithin and fatty acids. Very penetrating. Nourishing for dry, dehydrated skin, eczema and rough, scaly spots on sun-damaged skin (solar keratosis).
borage seed oil	Highest source of gamma linoleic acid (GLA), which is good for ageing skin, psoriasis and eczema.
coconut oil	Recommended for hair care products as it adds shine to hair. Good for dryness, itching and sensitive skin. Makes a great cleanser.
evening primrose oil	Contains vitamins, minerals and GLA. Use for psoriasis, eczema, aged skin and scarring.
jojoba oil (wax)	Contains proteins and minerals. Mimics sebum, very penetrating. Great for nourishing skin. Also good for acne-prone and oily skin, as it helps dissolve excess sebum. Great in hair care products.
kukui nut oil	For all skin types. High in linoleic acid and oleic acid. This oil is wonderful for cosmetics and it gives a lovely, silky feeling to creams. If you can, buy it. Excellent penetration and is very moisturizing. Helps to prevent scarring. Contains sunscreen properties; however, a 30+SPF sunscreen should be used if your skin is exposed to the sun for long periods.
macadamia nut oil	Good for aged or dry skin. Contains Omega 5 and Omega 6 fatty acids. Softens skin and helps to maintain the skin's water balance.
olive oil	Contains protein, minerals and vitamins. Good for hair care, nail care, inflamed skin and acne.

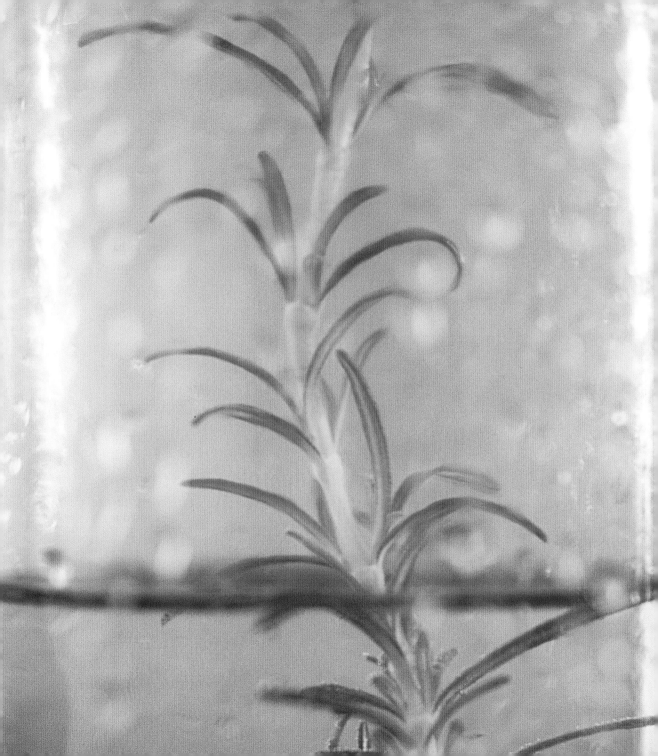

rose hip oil	Contains GLA. Good for dry or over-pigmented skin. Great for scars and ulcers. Do not use on acne-prone or oily skin.
sesame oil	For all skin types. Contains vitamins and is a particularly good source of vitamin E. Also contains minerals, proteins and amino acids.
soya bean oil	For all skin types, particularly acne-prone and oily skin. Good source of protein, minerals and vitamin E. Use carefully on sensitive skin and do not use if you have allergies to soya products.
sweet almond oil	For all skin types. Helps to relieve itching dryness. This oil is rich in protein.
wheat germ oil	Contains protein, minerals and vitamins. Good for stretch marks, prematurely aged skin, eczema and psoriasis. Do not use if you have a wheat or gluten allergy.

ESSENTIAL OILS

Essential oils should be used with caution. Keep oils out of the reach of children, as most oils are lethal if drunk, even in small amounts. Essentials oils are highly concentrated and when used on the body, they should always be diluted with a carrier oil, such as apricot kernel, jojoba, sweet almond or grapeseed oils. There are many essential oils that are unsafe to use during pregnancy. Check with a naturopath or doctor before using essential oils.

As a guideline, the essential oil content in skincare products would be:

- 1.5% for face creams;
- 2.5% for body creams;

- 3% for foot creams;
- 1% for products used during pregnancy; and
- 1% for hair care products (as the scalp is more sensitive than the skin on the rest of the body).

These are just a few essential oils to choose from:

benzoin	Reduces inflammation and soothes the skin. Also helps to reduce skin irritations.
carrot seed	Good for dryness, dermatitis, ageing skin and eczema.
chamomile, German	Helps reduce inflammation. Calming. Good for acne and allergies. Also good for rosacea, which is a chronic inflammation of the skin, that causes redness and pimples.
frankincense	Effective in healing wounds. Good for mature, ageing skin and wrinkles.
geranium	Balances and tones the skin.
jasmine	Softening. Smoothing. Helps to improve skin elasticity.
juniper	A great detoxifier. Helps combat cellulite and acne.
lavender	For all skin types. Soothes itchy skin. Good for acne, bruises, burns and warts.
lemon	Works on connective tissue. Good detoxifier. A great oil to use in hand and nail care products.

myrrh	Cooling. Helps reduce inflammation. Good for mature skin.
neroli	Good for sensitive skin. Also helps with scarring and thread veins.
palmarosa	Great in all skincare products. Hydrates and moisturizes the skin.
patchouli	Great for cracked skin, sores, skin allergies and mature skin.
rose	Particularly good for dry, mature and sensitive skin. Helps inflammation.
rosewood	Promotes cellular regeneration. Good for sensitive or inflamed skin.
sandalwood	For all skin types, particularly dry, dehydrated skin.
tea tree	Good for all infected wounds and ingrown hairs.
ylang-ylang	Balances skin sebum. Good in hair care products.

OTHER INGREDIENTS

aloe vera gel	An emollient, which has moisturizing, soothing, softening and anti-inflammatory properties. Also contains an astringent action that is good for irritated skin. Can lessen sunspots over time.
borax	A naturally powdered mineral salt. IMPORTANT: Recipes containing borax should not be used for infants and children, pregnant women or those with sensitive skin.

coconuts	Coconut milk is used for skin softening, cleansing and soothing. Grated coconut husk can be used as a face scrub. Chopped coconut pulp can be used as a face scrub or mask.
coffee	Leftover ground coffee makes a great body scrub.
cucumber	Used for soothing, cooling, moisturizing and toning the skin.
ginger	Good for stiff, sore muscles. Rejuvenates and regenerates.
glycerine (vegetable)	A humectant. Helps to retain moisture in the skin.
lemon grass	Has antiseptic properties. Helps to clear skin and is a good face scrub. Also works as a natural insect repellent.
rice	Can be used as a natural body scrub.
rice flour	Used to soften, soothe or smooth the skin.
sea salt	Makes a great body scrub. A good detoxifier.
soya milk or powder	Can be used as a cleanser or mask.
tamarind powder	High in alpha hydroxy acid (AHA). Contains vitamin C. Brightens and smoothes skin. A good face peel.
turmeric powder	Antibacterial. Helps sooth, calm and cleanse. A natural moisturizer.

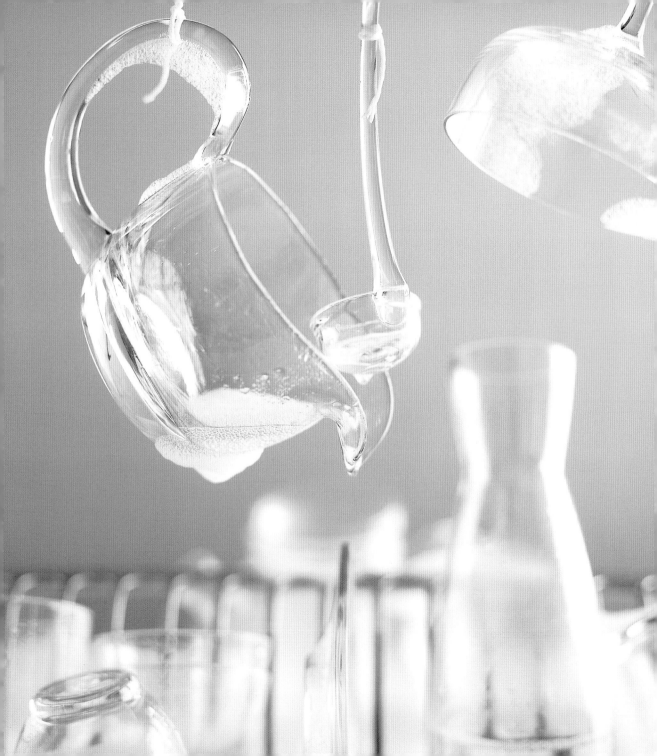

EQUIPMENT AND UTENSILS

When preparing skincare recipes, always wash your hands first and, if possible, use disposable gloves. All pans, whisks, spatulas, bowls, containers and other tools should be cleaned in hot soapy water, with a few drops of tea tree or lemon essential oil to minimize bacterial growth.

There are a few different ways to sterilize your containers:
- Run them through the dishwasher.
- Put them in the oven for 20 minutes at 120°C (235°F/Gas 1/2).
- Soak them in hot soapy water with some essential oils, such as lavender, lemon or tea tree, or you can use bleach.

Listed below are some basic utensils you will need:
- blender or whisk;
- bowls, preferably glass, a variety of sizes;
- coffee grinder for nuts, seeds and flowers when making scrubs;
- double boiler to melt wax, shea butter, cocoa butter and other hard waxes;
- mortar and pestle for crushing seeds, nuts and for mashing fruit;
- grater for grating fruit, etc;
- measuring jugs, 50 ml to 1 litre (13/4–35 fl oz);
- measuring vials, 20–45 ml (1/2–11/2 fl oz);
- scales — kitchen or electric;
- disposable gloves;
- funnel;
- eye dropper;
- strainer, to strain any fruit mash when collecting juices;
- spatulas — try to find spatulas that are not too hard or too soft and keep a variety of sizes;
- piping (icing) bags — for filling containers;
- glass containers are preferable to plastic, as essential oil properties may react with and permeate the plastic and can be destroyed; and
- measuring spoons.

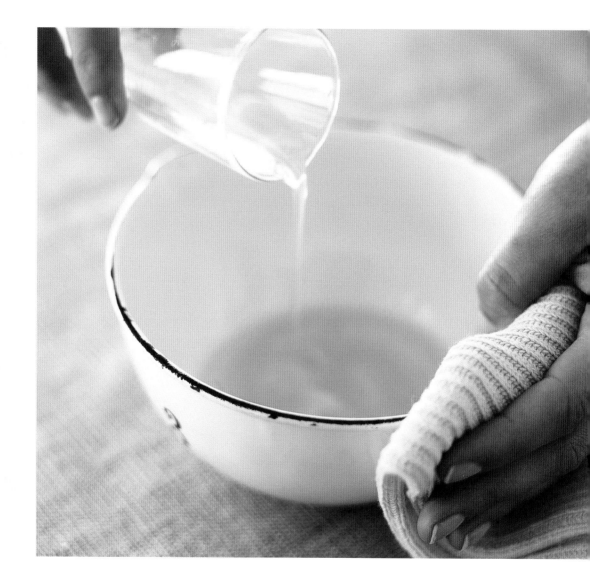

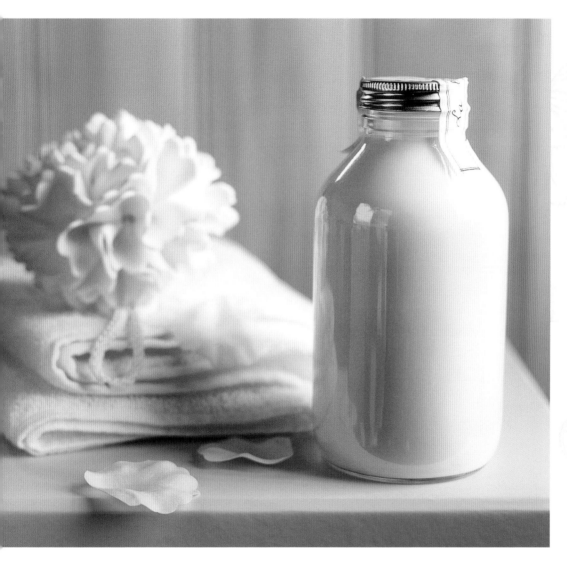

face care

cleansers

Make these face care cleansers in small quantities and store them in the refrigerator for absolute freshness.

coconut and olive cleanser

dry/combination/normal skin

This gentle cleanser will keep for a long time in the refrigerator. Refrigeration is essential in warm weather, as otherwise the cream will be very runny.

ingredients

45 ml (1^1/2 fl oz) coconut oil

10 g (^{1}/4 oz) cocoa butter

1^1/2 tablespoons light olive oil

25 ml (^{3}/4 fl oz) macadamia oil (or sweet almond oil)

20 drops essential oil of your choice

method

Melt the coconut oil and cocoa butter together very gently in a saucepan, taking care not to overheat. Stir to mix. Allow to cool a little.

Add the olive oil and macadamia oil and mix well. Cool a little, then add the essential oil and mix thoroughly. Pour into pots.

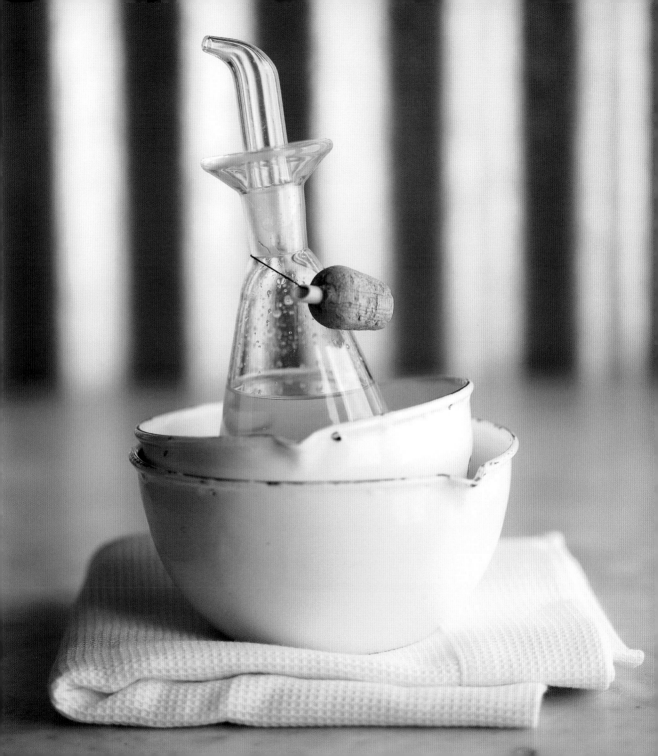

coconut honey cleansing cream

dry/normal skin

Store in the refrigerator, as coconut oil becomes liquid at room temperature.

ingredients

70 ml (2¼ fl oz) coconut oil

20 ml (½ fl oz) light olive oil (or grapeseed oil)

2 teaspoons distilled water

1½ teaspoons runny honey

10 drops essential oil of your choice (optional)

method

Melt the coconut oil and olive oil in the top half of a double boiler until liquid, taking care not to overheat. Remove from the heat. Warm the water and honey to the same temperature as the oil.

Slowly drizzle the water and honey into the oil, beating until no drops of water or honey can be seen. Cool slightly and add the essential oil, if desired. Beat to emulsify as the mixture cools. Pour into pots.

honey and peppermint cleansing jelly

normal/oily/combination skin

ingredients

1 heaped teaspoon powdered gelatine

1 teaspoon powdered pectin (or tragacanth)

135 ml (4$^1/_2$ fl oz) hot distilled water

2 teaspoons runny honey

55 ml (1$^3/_4$ fl oz) vegetable glycerine

70 ml (2$^1/_4$ fl oz) liquid Castile soap

$^1/_2$ teaspoon tincture of benzoin

20 drops peppermint essential oil

method

Mix the gelatine and pectin together well. Sprinkle over the hot water and stir until dissolved. Add the remaining ingredients. Bottle while still warm, shaking the jelly occasionally until the mixture is cold.

To use, massage the jelly gently into wet skin, then rinse off thoroughly. Pat your skin dry.

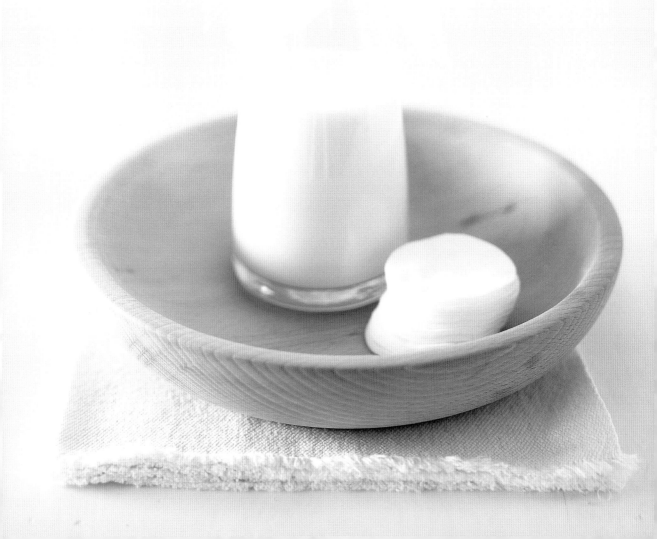

quick milk cleanser

dry/oily skin

For a good 'quickie' cleanser, use milk — full cream (whole) milk for dry skin, skimmed milk for oily skin — wiped on with a cottonwool ball. There is no need to wash the milk off, as it won't smell and will leave a natural sheen on your skin.

If you would like to refine this recipe you can add a handful of elderflower blossoms and 1 tablespoon yoghurt to 125 ml (4 fl oz/½ cup) milk. Heat to just below boiling and leave covered for half an hour. Strain through a fine sieve and then use.

Milk is a wonderful cleanser for fine or dry skin and can also be used to remove face masks.

milk and honey cleanser

all skin types

This is a quickly stimulating cleanser. It removes dead skin, oil and grime.

ingredients

    1 teaspoon dried milk powder

    1 teaspoon finely ground almonds

    2 teaspoons runny honey

    $1/2$ teaspoon rosewater (optional)

    3 drops sweet almond oil

method

Mix all the ingredients together well.

To use, pat the mixture from the base of the neck up to the hairline (do not apply to the skin around your eyes). Massage gently into the skin. Leave for 10 minutes, then wash off with warm water.

honey skin cleanser

all skin types

ingredients

60 ml (2 fl oz/^{1}/$_4$ cup) runny honey

125 ml (4 fl oz/^{1}/$_2$ cup) vegetable glycerine

40 ml (1^1/$_4$ fl oz) liquid Castile soap

method

Mix together all the ingredients, then pour the mixture into a clean plastic squeezebottle.

To use, dampen your skin and massage a little of the cleanser over your face and throat. Rinse with lukewarm water, then pat your skin dry.

milk and honey soap

normal/combination/oily skin

If you have normal, combination or oily skin, you may prefer to use soap to cleanse your face and neck. The glycerine and honey in this recipe are both humectants, which means that they attract moisture to the skin and hold it there.

ingredients

375 g (13 oz/4^1/$_2$ cups) finely grated, unscented
   pure soap or soap scraps
20–30 ml (^{1}/$_2$–1 fl oz) milk
2 teaspoons vegetable glycerine
2 teaspoons runny honey
20 drops rosemary essential oil
10 drops lavender essential oil
10 drops peppermint essential oil

method

Put the grated soap and milk in a heatproof bowl over a saucepan of simmering water, taking care that the base of the bowl does not touch the water. Stir occasionally until melted. If the mixture is too thick, add more milk and reheat. Use the least amount of milk possible, or the soap will shrink a lot as it dries. Add the glycerine and honey and stir until completely incorporated into the mixture. Allow to cool slightly, then add the essential oils.

Press the soap into moulds (such as soap dishes, individual jelly moulds, milk cartons cut in half, little baskets lined with muslin, etc), or shape it into balls. Set aside in an airy place to dry for 2–6 weeks. When the soap has hardened, you might like to polish it. Lightly moisten a cloth with some water to which a drop or two of essential oil has been added, then buff the soap.

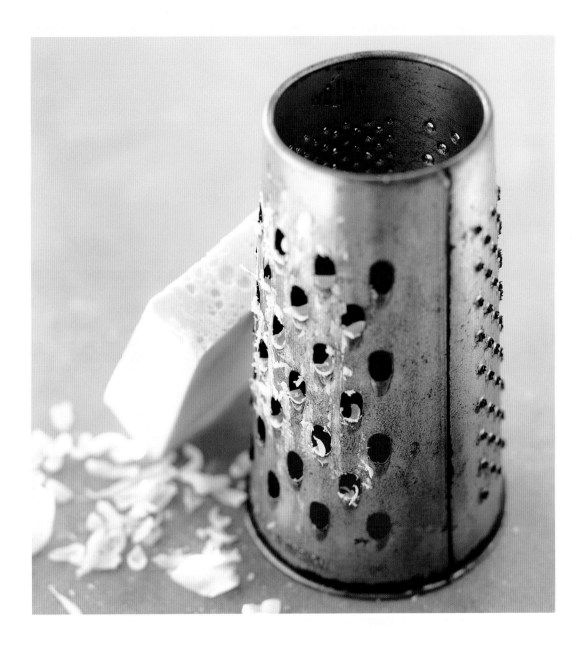

orange and honey cleansing cream

dry/normal skin

This lovely cleanser can also be used as a light moisturizer.

ingredients

10 g (¹/₄ oz) grated beeswax
30 ml (1 fl oz) sweet almond oil
20 ml (¹/₂ fl oz) coconut oil
2 teaspoons jojoba oil
30 ml (1 fl oz) distilled water
1 tablespoon orange juice
5 drops ylang-ylang essential oil
10 drops palmarosa essential oil
1 tablespoon honey

method

Combine the beeswax, sweet almond, coconut and jojoba oils in a heatproof bowl over a saucepan of boiling water, taking care that the base of the bowl does not touch the water. Stir constantly until the beeswax has melted.

Add the distilled water, 1 teaspoon at a time, while beating the mixture with a whisk or electric beater until it reaches a creamy consistency. Add the orange juice and keep beating until the cream thickens. Add the essential oils and honey and mix well. Spoon into glass containers.

gentle cleansing gel

all skin types, including sensitive, inflamed and acne-prone skin

ingredients

100 ml (3^1/$_2$ fl oz) distilled water (or use half water,
   half witch hazel)

^{1}/$_4$ teaspoon pectin (or xanthan gum)

20 g (^{3}/$_4$ oz) aloe vera gel

30 drops ylang-ylang essential oil

6 drops sandalwood essential oil

method

Heat the water over a very low heat. Sprinkle the pectin over the water. Use a whisk to blend to a smooth gel. If you prefer a smoother consistency, push the gel through a strainer.

Add the aloe vera gel and essential oils and mix well. Spoon into containers.

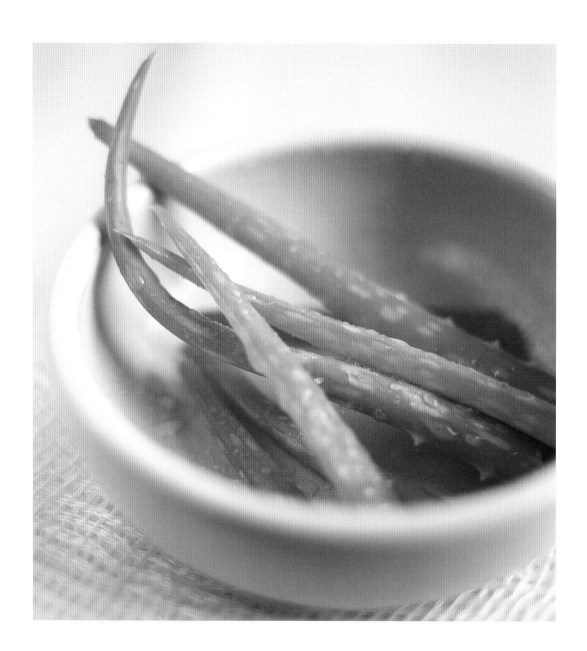

avocado and aloe vera cleansing oil

all skin types, particularly dry, irritated skin

ingredients

55 ml (1³/4 fl oz) jojoba oil

20 ml (¹/2 fl oz) avocado oil

20 ml (¹/2 fl oz) sweet almond oil

2 teaspoons vitamin E oil

50 g (1³/4 oz) aloe vera gel

2 teaspoons vegetable glycerine

method

Pour the oils in a saucepan and warm over a very low heat. At the same time, heat the aloe vera gel and glycerine in another saucepan, stirring constantly. Remove from the heat and stir the two mixtures together until cool. Pour into bottles. If the mixture separates later, shake the bottle before use.

You can also add the following essential oils to this recipe, if desired:

For inflamed or acne-prone skin:

10 drops chamomile essential oil

6 drops carrot seed essential oil

8 drops lavender essential oil

For dry skin:

10 drops sandalwood essential oil

5 drops geranium essential oil

8 drops rosewood essential oil

Aloe vera has moisturizing, soothing and anti-inflammatory properties.

washing water

sensitive/acne-prone/problem skin

Use this cleansing water to wash your face if your skin is very sensitive, or if you are troubled with acne or other skin problems. This water may also be used as a moisturizing lotion with the addition of 1 teaspoon sweet almond, macadamia or any other fine-textured oil.

ingredients

40 ml (1 1/4 fl oz) rosewater

60 ml (2 fl oz/1/4 cup) distilled water

1/4–1/2 teaspoon vegetable glycerine (try 1/4 teaspoon first
   and increase quantity to 1/2 teaspoon if you wish)

6 drops essential oil of your choice

method

Mix all the ingredients together in a 100 ml (3 1/2 fl oz) bottle and shake well until all ingredients are blended thoroughly. Leave for 4 days to synergize, shaking occasionally. Filter the mixture through coffee filter paper. Store in a dark-coloured glass bottle and shake well before use.

To use, take a palm-sized piece of cottonwool, dip it in warm water and squeeze it out well. Flatten it out into a pad, sprinkle with the Washing Water and use to cleanse the face and throat. Repeat if necessary. There is no need to use a toner after this treatment.

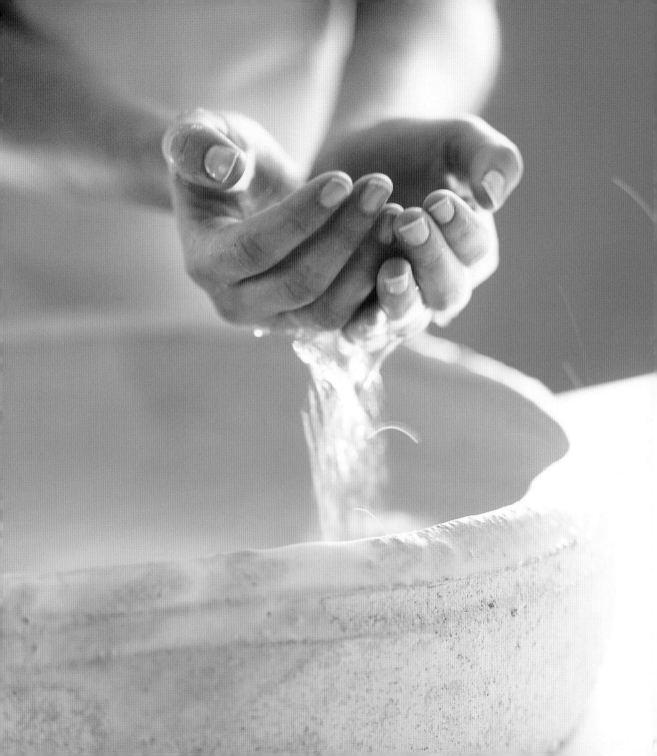

toners

Skin toners restore the acid mantle to your skin and leave it feeling fresh and clean. These preparations are also suitable for pre- and after-shave lotions.

To use, wet some cottonwool with water and squeeze it dry (this prevents any wastage of the lotion). Sprinkle the cottonwool with a few drops of the lotion and stroke it upwards over your throat and face.

rosewater and witch hazel toner

all skin types

The following is a simple but effective toner. If your skin is dry you can decrease the amount of distilled witch hazel and increase the amount of rosewater. If you have oily skin you can do the reverse.

ingredients

100 ml (3$\frac{1}{2}$ fl oz) rosewater (or hydrosol)
30 ml (1 fl oz) distilled witch hazel
$\frac{1}{2}$ teaspoon vegetable glycerine

method

Mix all the ingredients together, then pour into a bottle.

calendula skin toner

all skin types, particularly those troubled by spots or blemishes

This toner will keep in the refrigerator for up to 3 weeks, or it can be frozen in ice-cube trays and defrosted as needed.

ingredients

135 ml (4$\frac{1}{2}$ fl oz) boiling distilled water

2 teaspoons dried, crushed calendula flowers

20 drops tincture of benzoin

10 drops essential oil of your choice (optional)

method

Pour the boiling, distilled water over the dried calendula flowers, then cover and leave until cold. Strain through a sieve.

Add the remaining ingredients, mix well and leave to stand, covered, for 6–8 hours. Strain through coffee filter paper. Bottle or pour into ice-cube trays.

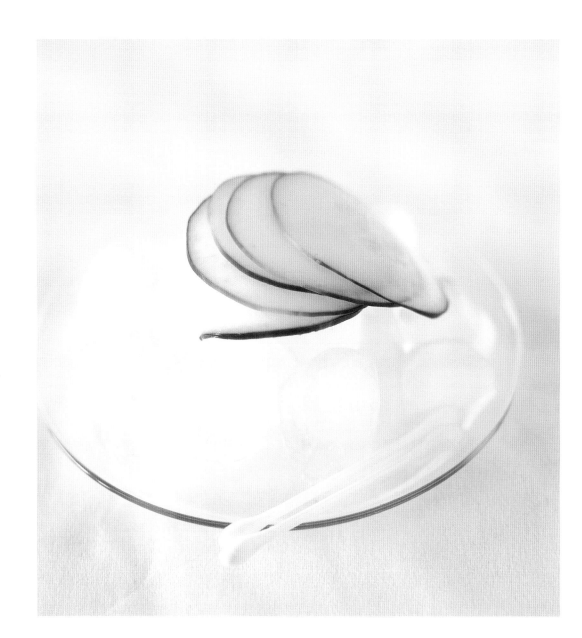

cucumber toner

all skin types, particularly inflamed skin

Cucumber toner doesn't keep well unless it is preserved. If you want to store it for a short time, say 7–21 days, use tincture of benzoin as a mild preservative. This toner can also be frozen in ice-cube trays and defrosted as needed.

ingredients

125 ml (4 fl oz/1/2 cup) cucumber juice
125 ml (4 fl oz/1/2 cup) distilled witch hazel
1 teaspoon tincture of benzoin

method

Mix all the ingredients together. Strain through a fine sieve and then through coffee filter paper. Bottle.

cucumber skin refresh

sensitive/inflamed skin

Juice one cucumber and combine with 25 ml (3/4 fl oz) distilled water and 2 teaspoons aloe vera gel. Mix thoroughly. Add 4 drops lavender essential oil and 2 drops frankincense essential oil and mix well. Pour into a bottle with a spray nozzle. Shake well.

Cucumber soothes the skin and contains both anti-itching and anti-inflammatory properties.

elderflower water

all skin types

This is a soothing, healing lotion for any kind of skin that has been in the wind and sun and is feeling dry and rough. It will keep for 2–3 weeks in the refrigerator, but can also be frozen in ice-cube trays and defrosted as needed.

ingredients

135 ml (4½ fl oz) boiling distilled water

2 teaspoons dried elderflower blossoms

1 teaspoon vegetable glycerine

20 drops tincture of benzoin

method

Pour the boiling, distilled water over the dried elderflowers, cover and allow to cool. Strain through a sieve.

Add the remaining ingredients, mix well and then leave to stand, covered, for 6–8 hours. Strain the mixture through coffee filter paper, then bottle.

neroli and lemon capillary toner

all skin types, most suitable for skin with broken capillaries

This recipe has a strengthening effect on thread veins, which are the tiny veins that appear most commonly on the cheeks, nose and legs.

ingredients

> 30 ml (1 fl oz) vegetable glycerine
> 20 g (3/4 oz) aloe vera gel
> 4 drops neroli essential oil
> 2 drops lemon essential oil

method

> Combine the vegetable glycerine and aloe vera gel. Add the essential oils and mix well. Spoon into airtight containers.

green tea toner

all skin types

A light spritzer full of anti-oxidants to protect and smooth the skin.

ingredients

1 pot freshly brewed green tea leaves,
   using 1 teaspoon leaves (2 teabags can be
   used if leaves are not available)
1 teaspoon honey
4 drops ylang-ylang essential oil (lavender or jasmine
   essential oil can be substituted, if preferred)

method

Strain the tea and pour into a bottle. Add the honey and ylang-ylang essential oil. Shake well.

Use morning and night.

Green tea is a powerful anti-oxidant. It reduces swelling and protects the skin.

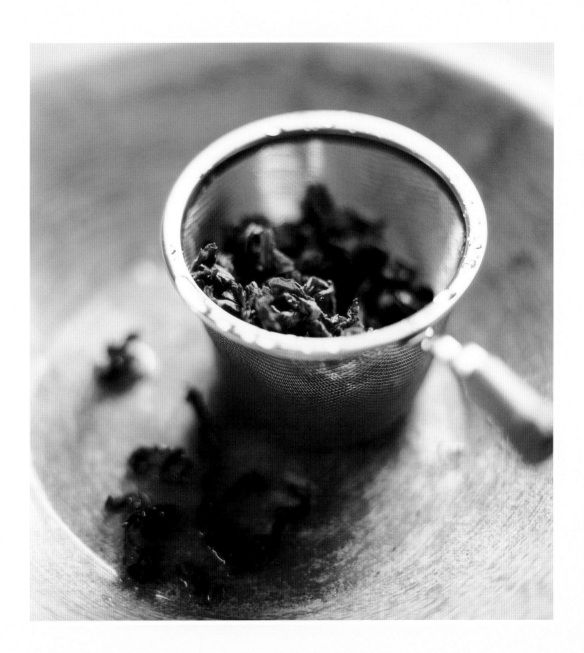

fragrant face spritzer

all skin types

ingredients

50 g (1³/4 oz/1 cup) rose petals

50 g (1³/4 oz/1 cup) frangipani flowers (or jasmine flowers)

55 ml (1³/4 fl oz) distilled water

30 ml (1 fl oz) aloe vera juice

method

Wash the rose petals and frangipani flowers. Pat dry and put into a food processor. Add the distilled water and aloe vera juice and process. Allow to sit for 1 hour.

Strain and pour into a bottle with a spray nozzle. Use as a toner or body spray.

floral spritzer

normal/oily skin

ingredients

50 g (1³/₄ oz/1 cup) rose petals (or frangipani flowers)

55 ml (1³/₄ fl oz) distilled water

25 ml (³/₄ fl oz) witch hazel

25 ml (³/₄ fl oz) aloe vera juice

1 teaspoon vegetable glycerine

method

Blend the rose petals and distilled water in a food processor. Leave to settle, then strain and discard the solids. Add the remaining ingredients.

Pour into a bottle with a spray nozzle. Use as a refreshing toner.

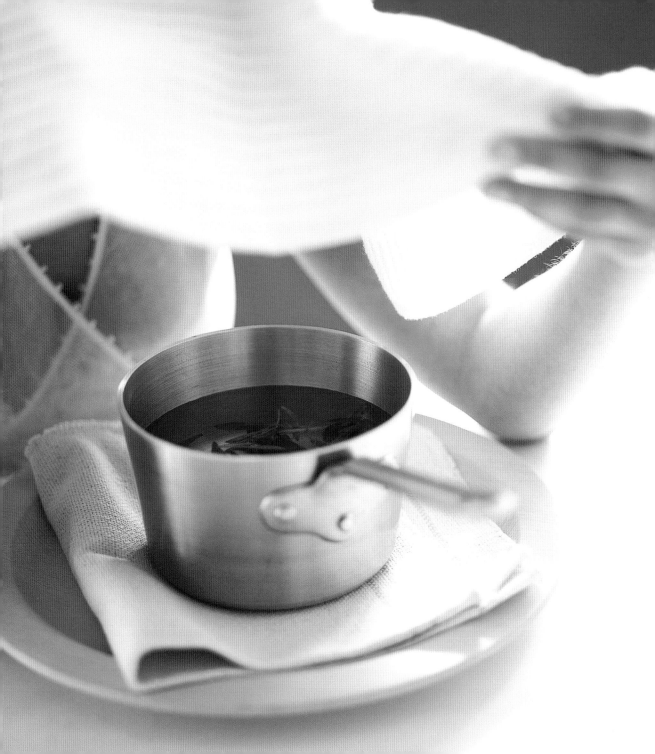

facial steaming

all skin types

Facial steaming causes the skin to perspire, which helps to deep-cleanse every pore. It also loosens grime and dead skin cells. The heat from the steam stimulates the blood supply and hydrates the skin, which will look and feel softer and more youthful.

If you have 'thread veins' on your cheeks, you need to be careful when steaming. Apply a thick layer of moisturizer or night cream over the veins and hold your face about 40 cm (16 inches) away from the steam, no closer. Don't steam more than once a fortnight. If your skin is dry and sensitive, apply a thin layer of honey on your face and throat before you steam. Keep your face 40 cm (16 inches) away from the steam. Don't steam more than once a fortnight. Normal, combination and oily skins may be steamed as often as twice a week.

Have ready a shower cap, a large towel and a heatproof pad for the table. Wash or otherwise cleanse your face. Put on the shower cap. Put 4 tablespoons finely chopped herbs in a saucepan, pour over 2 litres (70 fl oz/8 cups) cold water and cover the pan with a lid. Bring to the boil, reduce the heat and simmer gently for 5 minutes, then put the pan on the heatproof pad and remove the lid. Add the essential oils to the pan.

Form a tent with the towel over the pan and your head. Those with problem-free skin can keep their face 20 cm (8 inches) away from the steam, for 5–10 minutes. Deep grime will be drawn to the surface of the skin. Splash your face with cool (not cold) water and finish with a tonic or astringent and some moisturizer.

For facial steaming recipes, see pages 50–52.

A NOTE ON INGREDIENTS

Herbs and citrus peel should be dried and finely chopped or rubbed. Seeds should be dried and crushed, and roots dried and ground or finely chopped. Essential oils may be used alone or with dried or fresh herbs. Add the oils immediately before using the treatment. No more than 8 drops essential oil may be used in 2 litres (70 fl oz/8 cups) boiling water. To prepare these recipes, see the instructions on page 49.

herbal blend for dry skin

ingredients

> 5 g (1/8 oz/1/4 cup) dried chamomile flowers and leaves
>
> 15 g (1/2 oz/1 cup) dried clover blossoms
>
> 25 g (1 oz/1/4 cup) dried ground comfrey root*
>
> 35 g (11/4 oz/1 cup) dried comfrey leaves*
>
> 60 g (21/4 oz/1 cup) dried fennel seeds and leaves
>
> 25 g (1 oz/1 cup) dried violet leaves and flowers

* Comfrey is a restricted substance in some countries.

herbal blend for oily skin

ingredients

>   30 g (1 oz/1 cup) dried lemon grass
>
>   40 g (1$^{1}/_{2}$ oz/1 cup) dried lemon peel and leaves
>
>   25 g (1 oz/$^{1}/_{4}$ cup) dried liquorice root
>
>   80 g (2$^{3}/_{4}$ oz/1 cup) dried comfrey root and leaves*
>
>   5 g ($^{1}/_{8}$ oz/$^{1}/_{4}$ cup) dried peppermint leaves

herbal blend for normal/combination skin

ingredients

>   60 g (2$^{1}/_{4}$ oz/1 cup) dried fennel seeds and leaves
>
>   20 g ($^{3}/_{4}$ oz/$^{1}/_{2}$ cup) dried lemon peel and leaves
>
>   20 g ($^{3}/_{4}$ oz/1 cup) dried orange peel and leaves
>
>   20 g ($^{3}/_{4}$ oz/1 cup) dried lavender flowers and leaves

* Comfrey is a restricted substance in some countries.

For the blends below, mix all the ingredients together in a small bottle. Leave for 4 days to blend. To prepare and use these recipes, see the instructions on pages 49 and 50.

essential oil blend for combination skin

ingredients

70 ml (2¼ fl oz) sweet almond oil

8 drops geranium essential oil

6 drops palmarosa essential oil

6 drops lavender essential oil

essential oil blend for dry skin

ingredients

70 ml (2¼ fl oz) sweet almond oil

8 drops rosewood essential oil

8 drops palmarosa essential oil

4 drops rose or lavender essential oil

essential oil blend for oily skin

ingredients

80 ml (2½ fl oz) grapeseed oil

12 drops lemon essential oil

4 drops patchouli essential oil

4 drops sandalwood essential oil

You can dry your own citrus peel on wire cooling racks in a warm, well-aired position.

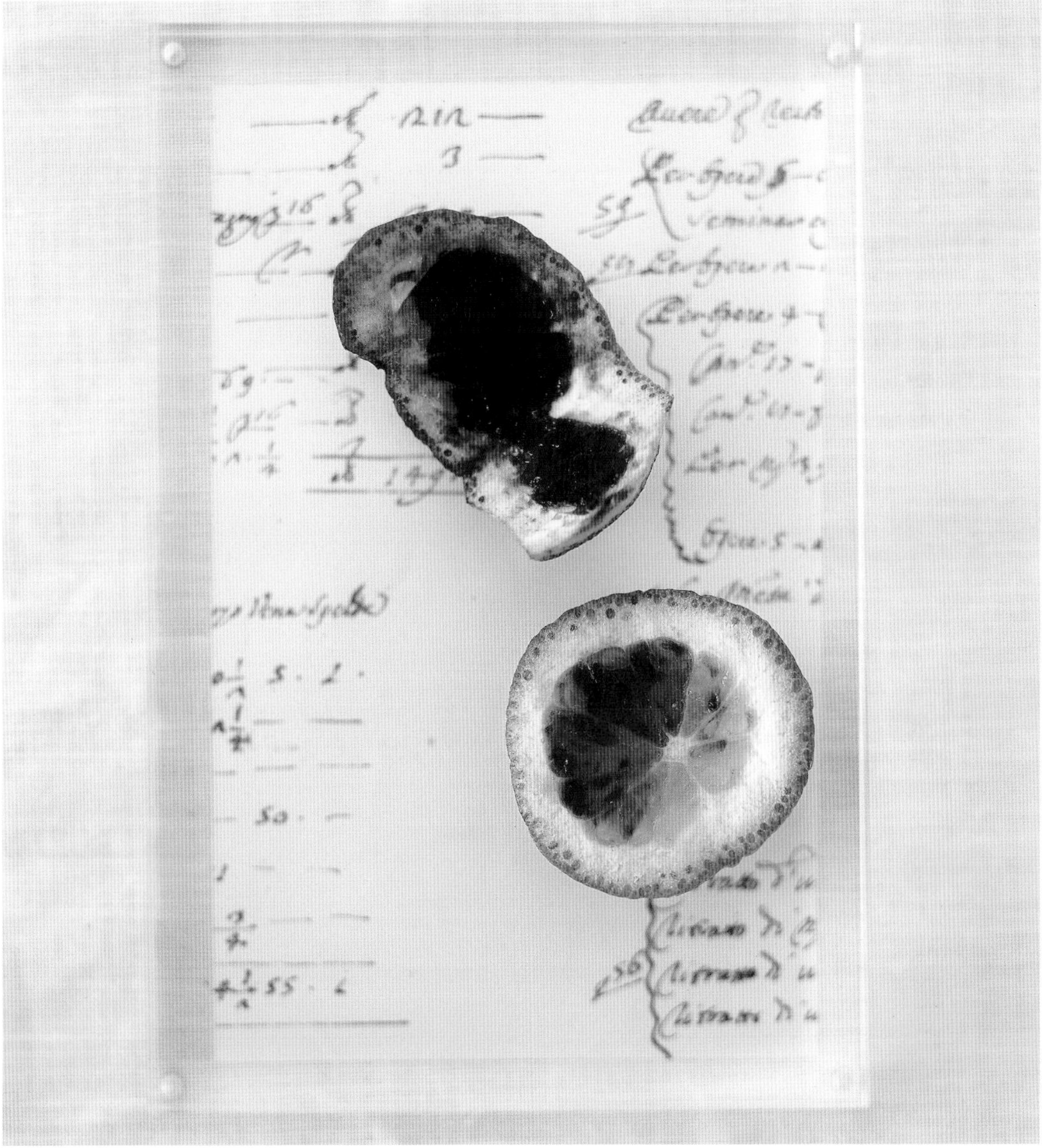

scrubs and masks

Scrubs and masks may be used for exfoliating, clearing excessive oiliness, refining pores, nourishing dry skin and improving circulation. Exfoliating the top layer of dead skin will enhance the performance of your moisturizers and serums, and give skin a smooth healthy complexion.

The frequency with which scrubs and masks can be used depends on your skin type. If you have oily or blemished skin you can use these preparations several times a week, but if your skin is fine and dry it would be wise to choose only the most gentle treatment and use it perhaps once a fortnight. Areas with obvious 'thread veins' should never be treated with masks or scrubs as the additional stimulation could worsen the condition.

Scrubs may be made in large quantities, stored in a glass jar in the bathroom and mixed as required. However, as most masks are made with fresh fruit, vegetables and milk or yoghurt, they should be prepared as needed or kept for no longer than 24 hours in the refrigerator.

parsley and lettuce scrub

all skin types

ingredients

2 parts powdered bran

2 parts powdered oatmeal

2 parts powdered soap

1 part dried parsley, powdered

1 part dried lettuce, powdered

1 part dried comfrey leaf, powdered*

method

Mix all the ingredients together. Store in an airtight jar.

To use, put 4 teaspoons in a small bowl. Add enough water or milk to form a soft paste and massage gently into your skin using small circular movements. Rinse off with cool water. Blot your skin dry with a soft towel.

* Comfrey is a restricted substance in some countries.

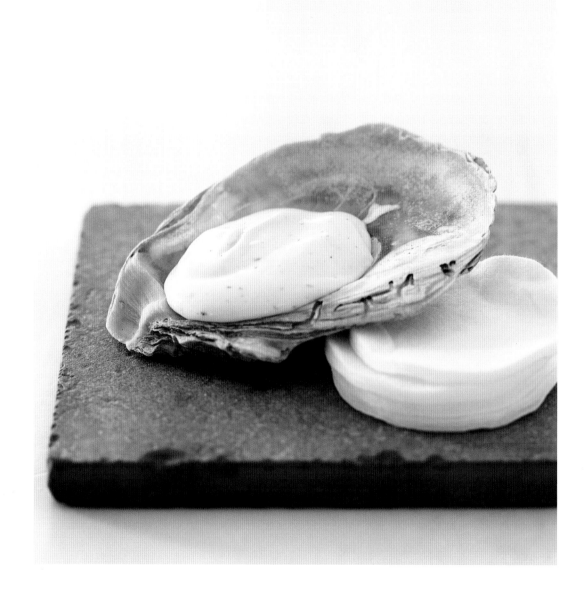

almond scrub

all skin types

This recipe is gentle enough to use as a regular cleanser, provided that the almonds are very finely ground.

ingredients

2 teaspoons sweet almond oil
4 teaspoons very finely ground almonds
1 teaspoon cider vinegar
1 drop lavender or palmarosa essential oil
distilled water

method

Mix all the ingredients to a smooth paste, adding distilled water as needed. To use, massage gently into your skin, rinse off with lukewarm water and pat your skin dry.

aromatic face scrub

all skin types

Slowly combine 3 tablespoons wheat bran with 1 tablespoon ground almonds, 1 tablespoon poppy seeds and 2 tablespoons dried lavender flowers (or dried chamomile). Juice one cucumber (or one apple) and add enough of the juice to the dry ingredients to form your preferred consistency. Mix well and spoon into a glass container.

Use the mask once a week if you have sensitive skin, and up to three times a week for normal to oily skin.

Almonds are very softening to the skin. Finely ground almonds and oatmeal thicken the scrubs, as well as refine the skin.

yoghurt and yeast scrub

normal/combination/oily skin

Yeast stimulates the circulation, bringing blood to the surface of the skin. Be very careful when using this scrub not to overstimulate the cheeks, where the delicate capillary veins lie near the surface. This recipe is sufficient for one treatment. It does not keep.

ingredients

4 teaspoons yoghurt

2 teaspoons ground almonds

1 teaspoon brewer's yeast

1 teaspoon runny honey

method

Mix all the ingredients together. Use the scrub immediately.

To use, gently massage the scrub onto your skin. Rinse off with lukewarm water, then pat your skin dry.

parsley and papaya quick fix

normal/oily/congested skin

This scrub is beneficial for congested skin and for a thick, uneven complexion.

ingredients

1 papaya
2 tablespoons dried rosehip tea leaves
1 tablespoon almonds, ground or chopped
2 tablespoons dried parsley

method

Cut the papaya in half, take out the seeds and dry them in the sun.

Juice the rest of the papaya. Combine 1/2 cup of the juice, the seeds and the remaining ingredients and mix into a paste. Use the scrub 1–2 times a week.

coconut and rice scrub

normal/dry skin

Combine 60 g (2 1/4 oz/1 cup) grated coconut with 30 g (1 oz) ground rice. Add 60 ml (2 fl oz/1/4 cup) coconut milk and 4 drops palmarosa essential oil and blend into a paste. Spoon into a glass container.

cinnamon and lemon grass face scrub

all skin types

This scrub gently removes dead skin cells, leaving your skin smooth and fresh.

ingredients

15 g (^{1}/2 oz/^{1}/4 cup) dried lemon grass

2 tablespoons ground cinnamon

distilled water

2 drops juniper essential oil

1 drop ylang-ylang essential oil

method

Crush the lemon grass, using a mortar and pestle, and combine with the cinnamon. Add enough distilled water to form a paste. Add the essential oils and mix thoroughly. Use 1–3 times a week.

ginseng and lemon grass skin renewal

all skin types, beneficial for acne-scarred skin

ingredients

3 tablespoons white clay

3 tablespoons Korean ginseng tea leaves

3 tablespoons dried lemon grass, crushed

distilled water (or witch hazel)

method

Combine the dry ingredients. Slowly add enough of the water to form a paste. Spoon into a glass jar. Gently scrub your face 2–3 times a week. Wash off with lukewarm water, then moisturize.

Lemon grass has antiseptic properties and helps to clear the skin.

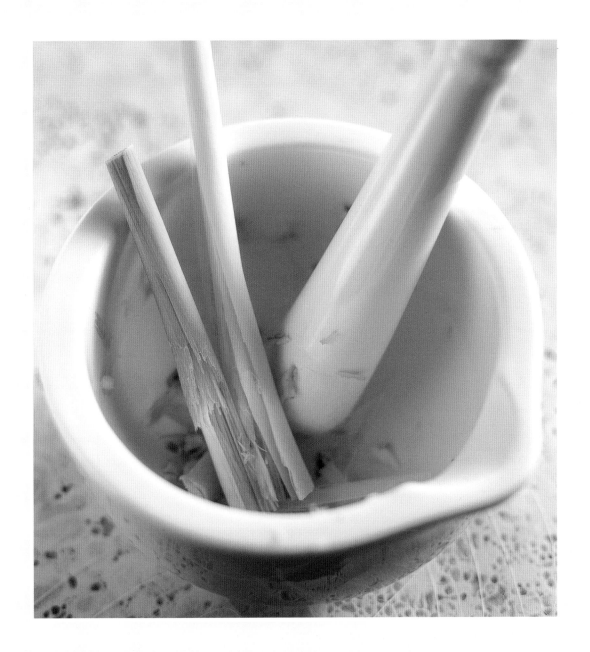

detox complexion mask

normal/oily/congested skin

The combination of the two clays helps to rebalance oil flow and strengthen the skin cells.

ingredients

30 g (1 oz) green clay (if green clay is not available,
   use 60 g white clay)

30g (1 oz) white clay

10 g ($^{1}/_{4}$ oz) tamarind powder

30 ml (1 fl oz) witch hazel (or distilled water)

4 drops juniper essential oil

4 drops lavender essential oil

method

Combine all the dry ingredients. Slowly add the witch hazel and blend to a paste.
Add the essential oils and mix thoroughly.

To use, apply to your face, avoiding the eye area. Keep the mask wet by spraying with
water or face toner. Leave the mask on for 10–15 minutes, then wash off with lukewarm water.

chamomile soothing mask

sensitive/dry/inflamed skin

ingredients

30 g (1 oz/$^1/_2$ cup) soya beans

90g (3$^1/_4$ oz/$^1/_2$ cup) rice flour

2 teaspoons chamomile tea leaves, brewed
    in $^1/_4$ cup boiling water

2 teaspoons honey

method

Soak the soya beans for 20–30 minutes in water, then drain. Blend in a food processor. Add the rice flour and chamomile tea and mix to a paste. Add the honey and mix well. To use, spread on your face and leave for 10 minutes. Wash off with lukewarm water.

grape mask

normal/oily skin

Make a paste of 2 teaspoons cornflour (cornstarch) and 2 tablespoons chamomile-infused tea. Mash 10 grapes, then combine with the paste and mix well.

To use, apply to your face and leave for 15 minutes. Wash off with lukewarm water, then apply moisturizer.

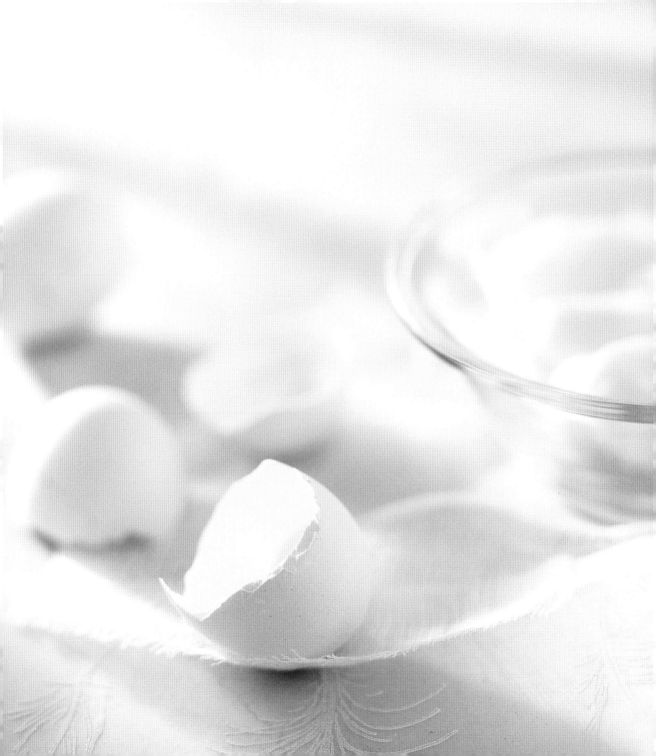

quick egg mask

all skin types

An egg white lightly beaten, smoothed on the skin and rinsed off after 20 minutes, will tighten and tone your skin. If your skin is dry, smear some honey or oil on your skin before spreading on the egg white. If you have oily skin, $1/2$ teaspoon lemon juice may be beaten into the egg white.

quick honey mask

all skin types

A simple honey mask is a stimulating cleanser and can be done very quickly, easily and cheaply. Spread some warm, runny honey over your face and very gently begin to tap your skin with your fingertips until there is a feeling of 'pulling'. This takes about 2 minutes. Stop tapping and rinse your face well with coolish water. Blot dry.

Egg white helps to smooth and tighten the skin.

basic mask

all skin types

Make a basic mask in advance and store it in an airtight container ready for mixing.

ingredients

100 g (3^1/$_2$ oz) white clay

25 g (1 oz) cornflour (cornstarch)

4 teaspoons very finely ground oats

4 teaspoons very finely ground almonds

method

Mix together all the ingredients and store in a tightly covered container.

To use, mix 4 teaspoons of the mask into a soft paste with honey, fruit juice or pulp, vinegar, egg, oil or herbal tea. Spread the mask over your face and neck (be very careful if you have dry skin or 'broken' veins, as masks may be overstimulating). Lie down on your bed or in the bath and relax for 15–20 minutes. You could also place cucumber slices or cottonwool soaked in distilled witch hazel on your eyes. Wash the mask off with warm water and follow with a cool splash.

turmeric face saver

all skin types, particularly irritated skin

A gentle mask to soothe and cleanse the skin. White clay is the most gentle of clays. Turmeric is a natural moisturizer and an anti-irritant.

ingredients

2 tablespoons turmeric powder

2 tablespoons white clay (or rice flour)

4 drops of essential oil, such as rosewood, palmarosa
    or neroli (optional)

distilled water (or rice milk)

method

Combine the turmeric, clay and essential oil. Add enough distilled water to make a paste and mix well.

To use, apply over clean face. Leave on for 15–20 minutes, then wash off with lukewarm water.

egg and lemon mask

all skin types

This mask may be used as a cleanser if the wholemeal (whole-wheat) flour is replaced with arrowroot. It is a deep cleanser that will leave your skin feeling soft. If your skin is dry, replace the lemon juice with orange juice for a gentler action.

ingredients

1 egg white, beaten

1 teaspoon olive oil (or sweet almond oil)

2 teaspoons lemon juice (or orange juice)

4 drops lemon essential oil (or orange essential oil)

wholemeal (whole-wheat) flour, to thicken

method

Mix all the ingredients together and store in the refrigerator. Use within 3 days.

To use, spread the mask over your face and neck (be very careful if you have dry skin or 'broken' veins, as masks may be overstimulating). Lie down and relax for 15–20 minutes. Wash the mask off with warm water, then splash your face and neck with cool water.

Lemon stimulates the skin's connective tissue.

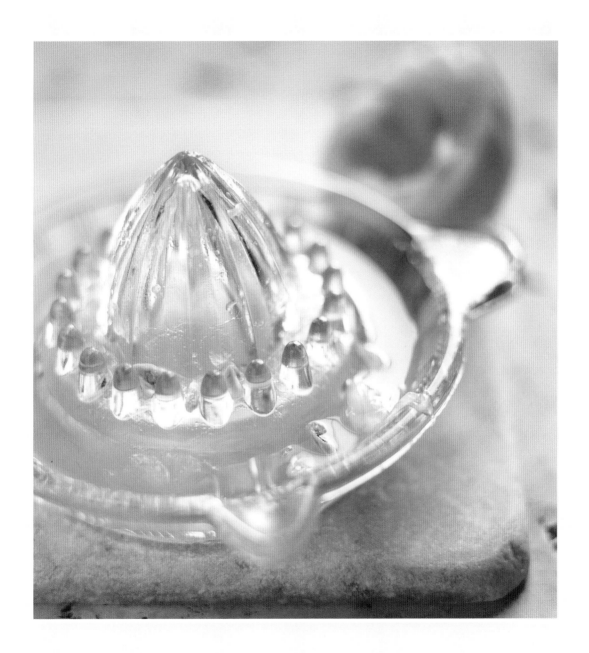

treatments

Many fruits can be used as alpha hydroxy acid (AHA) treatments, sloughing off dead skin cells to reveal a smooth complexion: pineapple is great for congested, oily, thick skin; guava is a good exfoliator; grapes hydrate the skin; kiwi fruit contains vitamin E; and apples are great for moisturizing the skin.

soy and linseed scrub and mask

all skin types

This two-in-one combination is great for a quick skin rescue!

ingredients

2 tablespoons linseed, sunflower and almond blend (LSA)

2 tablespoons rice flour

1 tablespoon honey

soya milk

method

Combine the LSA and rice flour (if you cannot find LSA, buy the items separately and crush together using a mortar and pestle). Add the honey and enough soya milk to make a paste and mix well.

To use, apply over your face and neck. You can use as a scrub or leave on for 15–20 minutes to hydrate and nourish your skin. Wash off with lukewarm water or milk.

yoghurt and avocado nourishing mask

all skin types

ingredients

1 ripe avocado

1 ripe banana

3 tablespoons plain yoghurt

$1/4$ teaspoon vitamin E oil

3 tablespoons aloe vera juice

method

Mash the avocado and banana to form a paste. Add the yoghurt and vitamin E oil and mix well.

To use, massage the mask into your skin. Soak a piece of gauze in the aloe vera juice and place the gauze over the mask to infuse the ingredients. Leave on for 10–20 minutes, then rinse off.

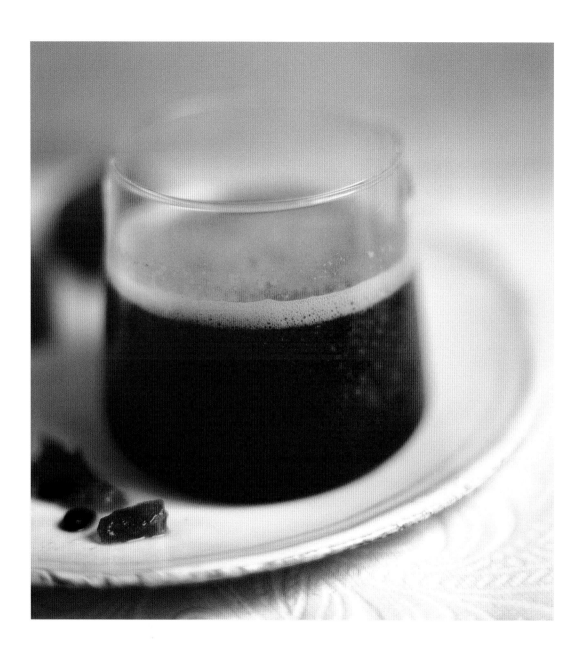

papaya and watermelon treatment

normal/oily/congested skin

ingredients

185 g (6^1/$_2$ oz/1 cup) peeled, seeded and chopped papaya

185 g (6^1/$_2$ oz/1 cup) peeled, seeded and chopped watermelon

method

Blend the papaya and watermelon in a food processor. Strain and discard any solid particles (these can be used in the garden as compost). Use the remaining juice as a face mask (leave on for 10 minutes, then rinse), or as a toning solution using cottonwool (leave on the skin, no need to rinse off).

ginseng and honey quick fix

all skin types

This is a great instant lift, which is both hydrating and soothing.

ingredients

2 tablespoons freshly brewed ginseng tea

3 tablespoons honey

2 drops carrot seed essential oil

method

Mix all the ingredients thoroughly and apply over clean skin. Leave on for 20 minutes. Wash off with warm water, then apply moisturizer.

Papaya pulp contains natural alpha hydroxy acids (AHAs). It cleanses and exfoliates the skin and is a good treatment for itchy skin, acne and psoriasis.

spot the blemish

blemished skin

ingredients

1 tablespoon turmeric powder

3 tablespoons white clay

40 ml (1^1/$_4$ fl oz) ginseng tea

40 ml (1^1/$_4$ fl oz) comfrey tea*

1 drop tea tree essential oil

1 drop lemon essential oil

method

Combine the turmeric powder and clay. Add the teas and blend to form a paste. Add the essential oils and mix thoroughly.

This brightly coloured blemish treatment can be used on pimples 1–3 times a day.

* Comfrey is a restricted substance in some countries.

blemish treatment

blemished skin

ingredients

  1 green teabag, brewed in $1/2$ cup boiling water

  4 drops chamomile tea (German or Roman)

  20 g ($3/4$ oz) white clay

  1 drop tea tree essential oil

  2 drops geranium essential oil

method

Add enough tea to the clay to form a paste. Add the essential oils and mix well. Apply to blemishes at night. Wash off in the morning with warm water or green tea.

gentle acne and blemish gel

blemished and acne-prone skin

ingredients

  2 teaspoons evening primrose oil

  20 g ($3/4$ oz) aloe vera gel

  2 drops juniper essential oil

  3 drops lavender essential oil

  1 drop tea tree essential oil

method

Add the evening primrose oil to the aloe vera gel and stir to combine. Add the essential oils and mix well. Apply to blemishes up to 3–4 times daily.

depigmentation gel

pigmented skin

Aloe vera gel is reputed to remove brown marks on the skin.

ingredients

50 g (1³/4 oz) aloe vera gel

2 tablespoons tamarind powder

40 ml (1¹/4 fl oz) raspberry leaf tea

10 drops lemon essential oil

8 drops carrot seed essential oil

4 drops parsley essential oil

method

Combine the aloe vera gel and the tamarind powder. Mix well. Add the raspberry leaf tea and blend thoroughly with a whisk. Add the essential oils, then mix well.

Apply daily for 6 months to the blemished areas.

Raspberry contains lactic acid, an alpha hydroxy acid (AHA). Raspberry whitens the skin and is good for removing brown skin spots.

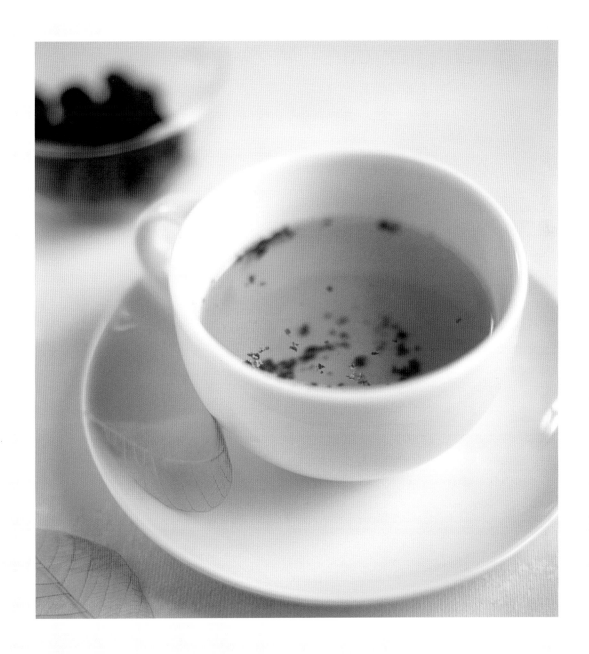

moisturizers

super hydrator

all skin types

ingredients

40 ml (1^{1}/4 fl oz) apricot kernel oil

20 ml (^{1}/2 fl oz) olive oil

1 tablespoon finely grated beeswax

^{1}/4 teaspoon borax*

60 ml (2 fl oz/^{1}/4 cup) distilled water (or rosewater)

1 tablespoon aloe vera gel

6 drops rosewood essential oil

4 drops lavender essential oil

4 drops frankincense essential oil

method

Gently melt the apricot kernel oil, olive oil and beeswax in the top half of a double boiler, stirring constantly. Combine the borax and distilled water in the top half of another double boiler and heat to the same temperature. Slowly add the oils and beeswax blend to the borax blend, stirring gently until the mixture has cooled to just warm.

Add the aloe vera gel and essential oils and mix well. Spoon into sterilized glass containers and store in a cool dark place.

* Recipes containing borax should not be used for infants and children, pregnant women or those with sensitive skin.

moisture defence

normal/dry skin

ingredients

Phase A

1 teaspoon vegetable glycerine

40 ml (1^1/$_4$ oz) distilled water (or rosewater)

1 teaspoon borax*

^{1}/$_2$ teaspoon vitamin E oil

Phase B

2 teaspoons grated beeswax

2 teaspoons cocoa butter

1 teaspoon rosehip oil

2 teaspoons sweet almond oil

2 teaspoons avocado oil

2 teaspoons jojoba oil

Phase C

8 drops rosewood essential oil

5 drops carrot seed essential oil

8 drops rose essential oil in 3% jojoba oil **

method

Gently melt Phase B ingredients in the top half of a double boiler. Stir until just melted. Combine Phase A ingredients in the top half of another double boiler and heat to the same temperature as Phase B. If the mixture thickens, reheat and stir gently. Remove from the heat and leave to cool for 10 minutes. Combine Phase A and Phase B ingredients. Add Phase C essential oils and mix thoroughly. Spoon into glass containers. Store in a cool place.

* Recipes containing borax should not be used for infants and children, pregnant women or those with sensitive skin.

** As rose is a very expensive essential oil and very little is required, it is often sold as 3% rose in jojoba (97%).

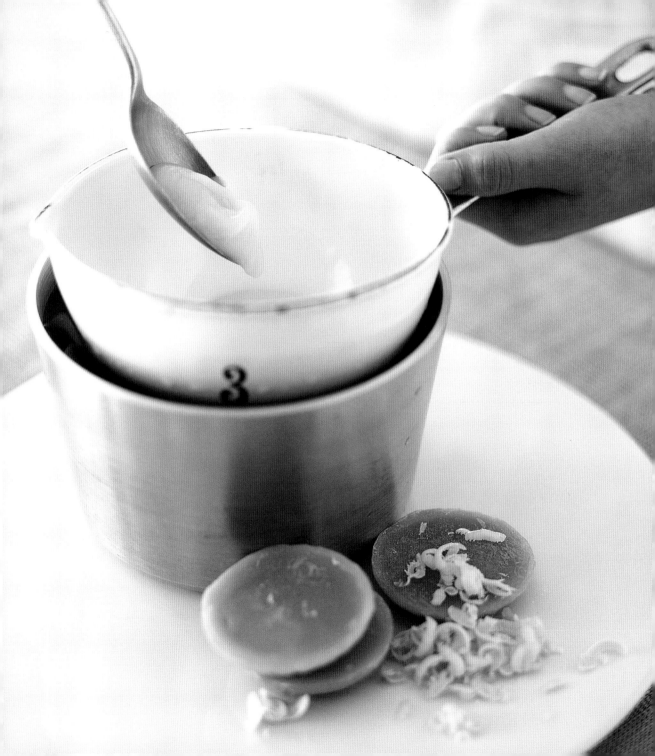

satin smooth moisture lotion

most skin types

This is a lovely, soft lotion that is so moisturizing it can double as a body oil. Store in the refrigerator and shake well before use.

ingredients

Phase A

150 ml (5 fl oz) distilled water

1/2 teaspoon borax*

50 drops grapefruit seed extract (optional preservative)

Phase B

1/2 teaspoon anhydrous lanolin

3 teaspoons finely grated beeswax

60 ml (2 fl oz/1/4 cup) sweet almond oil

40 ml (11/4 fl oz) light sesame or jojoba oil

Phase C

10 drops essential oil of your choice

method

Gently melt the ingredients for Phase B together in the top half of a double boiler. Stir until all the ingredients are melted but not overheated. Combine all the ingredients for Phase A and heat until the mixture is the same temperature as Phase B. Slowly trickle Phase A into Phase B, stirring constantly and reheating gently if the mixture begins to thicken. Remove from the heat and stir until the outside of the container feels just a little hotter than your hand. Add the Phase C essential oil and mix thoroughly. Spoon into sterilized containers.

* Recipes containing borax should not be used for infants and children, pregnant women or those with sensitive skin.

almond rose cream

dry/combination/normal skin

This moisturizing cream should be stored in the refrigerator.

ingredients

Phase A

60 ml (2 fl oz/$^1/_4$ cup) rosewater

1 teaspoon borax*

40 drops grapefruit seed extract (optional preservative)

Phase B

90 ml (3 fl oz) sweet almond oil

90 ml (3 fl oz) jojoba oil (or macadamia oil)

2 teaspoons finely grated, tightly packed beeswax

1000 IU vitamin E d'alpha tocopherol

Phase C

20 drops essential oil of your choice

method

Gently melt the ingredients for Phase B together in the top half of a double boiler (prick the vitamin capsules and squeeze out the contents). Stir until melted but not overheated. Combine the ingredients for Phase A and heat until the mixture is the same temperature as Phase B. Slowly trickle Phase A into Phase B, stirring constantly and reheating gently if the mixture begins to thicken. Remove from the heat. Stir until the outside of the container feels just a little hotter than your hand. Add the Phase C essential oil mix thoroughly. Spoon the cream into sterilized containers.

* Recipes containing borax should not be used for infants and children, pregnant women or those with sensitive skin.

protect and hydrate

all skin types, particularly sensitive skin

This sunscreen is not water-resistant. It has an SPF of 10. For extended periods in the sun, use a sunscreen with an SPF of 30 or above.

25 ml (3/4 fl oz) unrefined sesame oil
20 ml (1/2 fl oz) coconut oil
1 teaspoon calendula-infused oil
1/2 teaspoon vitamin E oil
6 drops lavender essential oil
3 drops ylang-ylang essential oil

method

Combine the ingredients in a dark bottle. Leave to synergize for 2–3 days. Apply every 2 hours.

lip balm

Melt 1 teaspoon finely ground beeswax with 1 teaspoon cocoa butter in the top half of a double boiler. Add 3 teaspoons olive oil, stir through then leave for 10 minutes to cool. Stir in 1/4 teaspoon each of vitamin E oil and honey. This recipe needs to be stirred quickly so the mixture doesn't set.

honey and vitamin rich night cream

dry skin

ingredients

Phase A

80 ml (2^1/$_2$ fl oz/^{1}/$_3$ cup) warm distilled water

1 teaspoon runny honey

Phase B

40 g (1^1/$_2$ oz) lanolin

1000 IU vitamin E d'alpha tocopherol

^{1}/$_2$ teaspoon sweet almond oil

5 drops carrot seed oil

^{1}/$_2$ teaspoon liquid lecithin

Phase C

6 drops lavender essential oil

2 drops patchouli essential oil

method

Gently melt the ingredients for Phase B together in the top half of a double boiler (prick the vitamin capsules and squeeze out the contents). Stir until all are melted but not overheated.

Combine Phase A ingredients and heat until the honey is melted and the temperature of the mixture is the same as Phase B. Slowly trickle Phase A into Phase B, stirring constantly and reheating gently if the mixture begins to thicken. Remove from the heat. Stir until the outside of the container feels just a little hotter than your hand. Add the Phase C oils and mix thoroughly. Spoon the cream into sterilized containers and store in the refrigerator.

Beeswax is a great moisturizing agent. It also emulsifies and thickens skincare preparations.

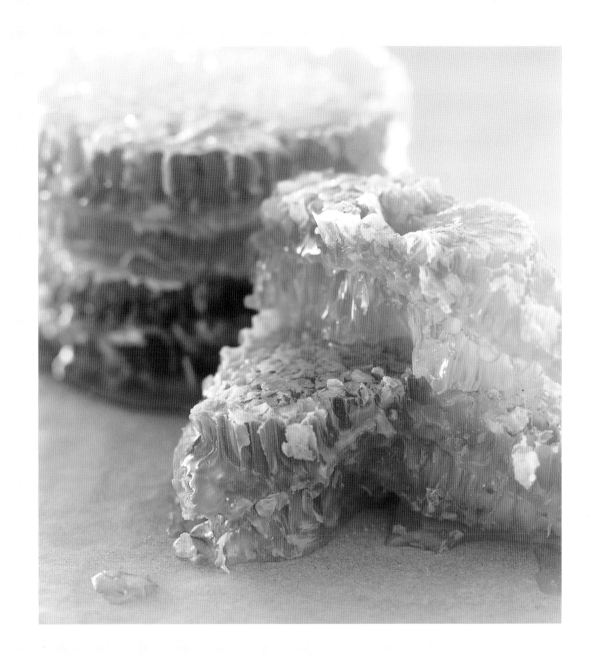

rescue elixir

all skin types

ingredients

3 tablespoons apricot kernel oil

1 tablespoon avocado oil

1 tablespoon jojoba oil

1 teaspoon vitamin E oil

5 drops neroli essential oil

3 drops myrrh essential oil

4 drops palmarosa essential oil

method

Combine all the ingredients in a dark bottle. Shake gently and, for best results, leave to synergize for 3 days.

Use the elixir on its own or under a moisturizer or mask.

anti-ageing oil serum

mature skin

This nourishing serum is packed with vitamins and minerals.

ingredients

60 ml (2 fl oz/$1/4$ cup) macadamia nut oil

2 teaspoons rosehip oil

2 teaspoons evening primrose oil

2 teaspoons jojoba oil

2 teaspoons borage seed oil (or wheat germ oil)

10 drops rosewood essential oil

5 drops sandalwood essential oil

5 drops carrot seed essential oil

5 drops lavender essential oil

$1/2$ teaspoon vitamin E oil

method

Combine all the ingredients in a dark bottle. Store in a cool, dark place. Leave the serum to synergize for 3 days.

The serum can be used on its own, as a moisturizer or under moisturizer, under night cream or under any face mask.

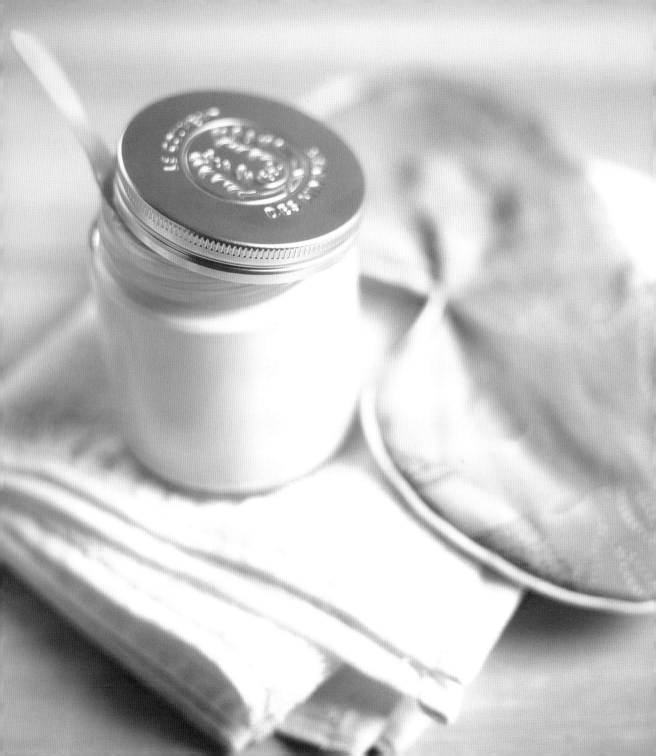

nourishing night cream

dry/sensitive/mature skin

ingredients

1 tablespoon finely grated beeswax

2 tablespoons jojoba oil

1 tablespoon evening primrose oil

1 tablespoon rosehip oil

1 teaspoon vitamin E oil

$1/4$ teaspoon borax*

40 ml ($1^1/4$ fl oz) rosewater (or distilled water)

6 drops sandalwood essential oil

2 drops geranium essential oil

2 drops carrot seed essential oil

2 drops patchouli essential oil

method

Heat the beeswax and the jojoba, evening primrose, rosehip and vitamin E oils in the top half of a double boiler, stirring constantly. At the same time, in the top half of another double boiler, mix the borax and rosewater and warm to around the same temperature.

Remove both mixtures from the heat and slowly add the oil blend to the water and borax blend, while stirring rapidly until the mixture reaches a creamy consistency. When the cream has cooled down to just warm, add the essential oils and stir well. Spoon into sterilized glass jars.

If your skin is very dry or stressed use a serum under the cream for maximum results.

* Recipes containing borax should not be used for infants and children, pregnant women or those with sensitive skin.

regenerating oil for dry skin

dry skin

ingredients

80 ml (2$^1/_2$ fl oz/$^1/_3$ cup) macadamia oil

1 teaspoon avocado oil

2 teaspoons evening primrose oil

2 teaspoons jojoba oil

1 teaspoon rosehip oil

15 drops palmarosa essential oil

5 drops lavender essential oil

5 drops sandalwood essential oil

5 drops ylang-ylang essential oil

method

Combine all the ingredients in a 100 ml (3$^1/_2$ fl oz) bottle. Shake well for several minutes. Leave for 4 days to blend. Store in a cool dark place.

Shake the bottle well before use. To use, gently massage the oil into slightly dampened skin. Use morning and night.

regenerating oil for normal skin

normal skin

ingredients

80 ml (2^1/$_2$ fl oz/^{1}/$_3$ cup) sweet almond oil

1 teaspoon avocado oil

1 teaspoon wheat germ oil

1 teaspoon jojoba oil

5 drops lavender essential oil

15 drops palmarosa essential oil

5 drops rosewood essential oil

5 drops sandalwood essential oil

method

Combine all the ingredients in a 100 ml (3^1/$_2$ fl oz) bottle. Shake well for several minutes. Leave for 4 days to blend. Store in a cool dark place.

Shake well before use. To use, gently massage the oil into slightly dampened skin.

regenerating oil for oily skin

oily skin

Those with oily skin will have noticed that there are areas on the face and neck which have little or no oil — these are mainly the throat, lips and under the eyes. Use this treatment on these areas but also use a thin smear over the whole face before going to bed, as the oils have the capacity to 'balance' and moisturize the skin without encouraging the oil glands to produce more sebum.

ingredients

80 ml (2$1/2$ fl oz/$1/3$ cup) grapeseed oil

2 teaspoons apricot oil

2 teaspoons evening primrose oil

10 drops bergamot essential oil

5 drops lemon essential oil

5 drops lavender essential oil

10 drops sandalwood essential oil

method

Combine all the ingredients in a 100 ml (3$1/2$ fl oz) bottle. Shake well for several minutes. Leave for 4 days to blend. Store in a cool dark place.

Shake the bottle well before use. To use, gently massage the oil into slightly dampened skin. Use morning and night.

If you have sensitive skin, you should check for an allergic reaction by testing a small amount of oil on the skin of your forearm.

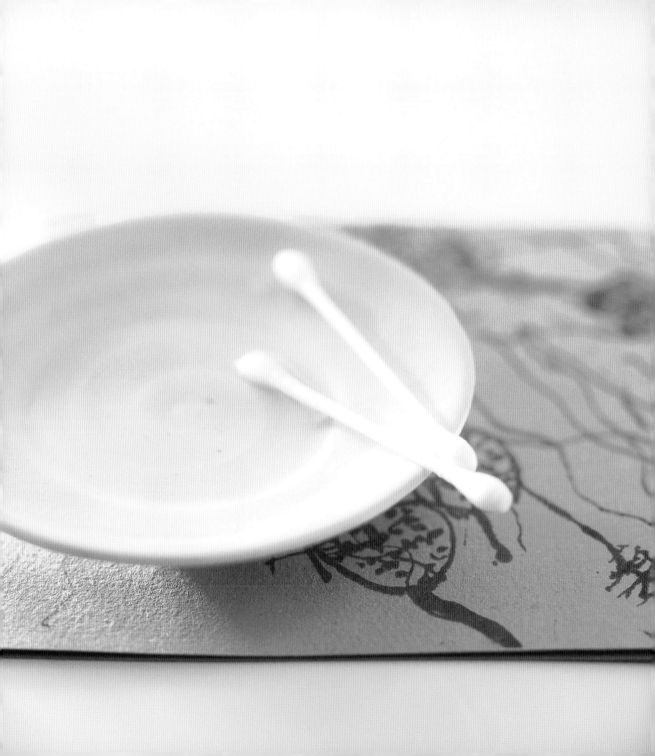

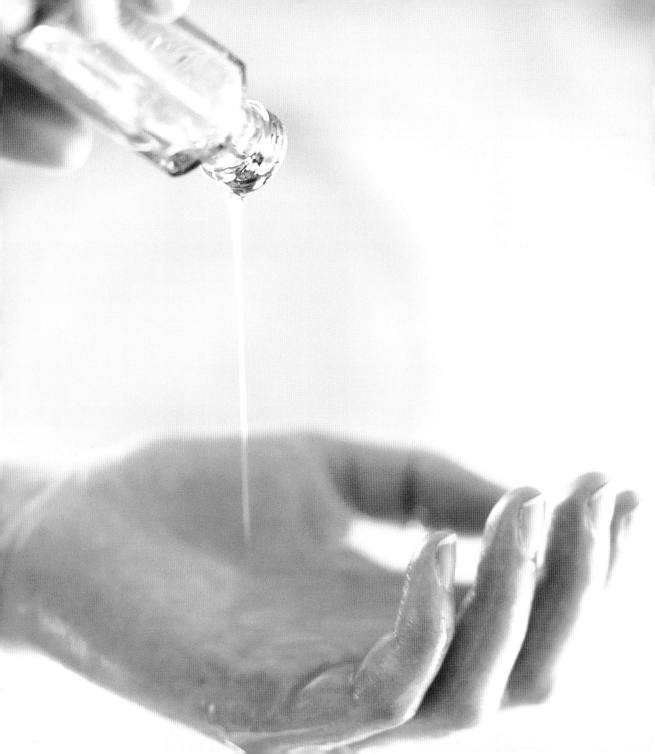

regenerating oil for the neck

dry/mature skin

The skin on the neck contains very few oil glands, so it needs a little more attention. This oil blend is very powerful and should be used at night to get the best result.

ingredients

2 teaspoons avocado oil

2 teaspoons evening primrose oil

55 ml (1³/4 fl oz) jojoba oil

4 teaspoons hazelnut oil

20 drops carrot seed oil

15 drops palmarosa essential oil

5 drops rosewood essential oil

5 drops frankincense essential oil

5 drops geranium essential oil

method

Combine all the ingredients in a 100 ml (3¹/2 fl oz) bottle. Shake well for several minutes. Leave for 4 days to blend. Store in a cool dark place.

To use, shake the bottle. Measure 5–10 drops into the palm of your hand and, with a light, upward motion, use the fingers of the other hand to spread the oil from the collarbones to the chin. Massage in, leave for 20 minutes, then blot the surplus off with a tissue.

When buying essential oils, check the label to see where the manufacturer sourced the ingredients, and if it runs checks for purity.

eye care

The thin, fine skin around the eyes shows early lines in the same way as the neck. It is super fragile and you can do more harm than good if you are heavy-handed. Use only the middle finger to gently pat creams and lotions on this area and avoid using heavy oils that can 'drag' the skin.

cucumber eye gel

all skin types

ingredients

20 g (3/4 oz) linseeds, crushed

150 ml (5 fl oz) boiling water

20 ml (1/2 fl oz) borage seed oil (or any fine-textured oil)

1 cucumber, juiced

2 drops carrot seed essential oil

method

Soak the linseeds in the boiling water overnight or simmer on the stove until a gel forms. Strain the seeds from the gel. Add the borage seed oil and mix well. Add the cucumber juice and stir. Add the carrot essential oil and stir thoroughly.

eye make-up remover

all skin types

Combine 30 ml (1 fl oz) castor oil with 30 ml (1 fl oz) light olive oil and mix well. To use, apply the mixture with a tissue or cottonwool ball to remove make-up from around the eyes. Follow with your regular face cleansing routine.

aloe vera eye gel

all skin types

ingredients

1 teaspoon borage seed oil

1 teaspoon evening primrose oil

30 g (1 oz) aloe vera gel

$1/4$ tablespoon vitamin E oil

5 drops lavender essential oil

method

Slowly add the borage seed and evening primrose oils to the aloe vera gel, stirring constantly. Add the vitamin E oil and lavender essential oil and stir. More aloe vera gel may be added if a thicker consistency is required.

To use, pat the gel gently around the eye area, morning and night.

coconut eye cleanser

all skin types

Combine 30 ml (1 fl oz) coconut oil with 30 ml (1 fl oz) macadamia nut oil and mix well. To use, apply to cottonwool and gently wipe the eye area.

around-the-eyes oil

all skin types

ingredients

55 ml (1³/4 fl oz) hazelnut oil

15 drops jojoba oil

35 drops evening primrose oil

15 drops carrot seed oil

1000 IU vitamin E d'alpha tocopherol

method

Put all the ingredients in a 55 ml (1³/4 fl oz) bottle (prick the vitamin capsules and squeeze the contents into the bottle). Shake the bottle well to mix and leave for 4 days to blend. Store in a cool dark place. Shake the mixture well before use. One drop under each eye should be enough. Apply the oil at night, leave it for 10 minutes and then carefully blot the excess off with a tissue. Avoid getting the oil into the eye itself or it will sting and could be harmful.

gentle eye oil

all skin types

Combine 2 teaspoons evening primrose oil, 1 teaspoon borage seed oil and 20 drops calendula-infused oil in a 20 ml (¹/2 fl oz) bottle and shake well. You may add 2–3 drops essential oils, such as carrot seed oil. One drop of oil should be sufficient to use around the eyes.

Avoid using too much oil on the skin around the eyes.

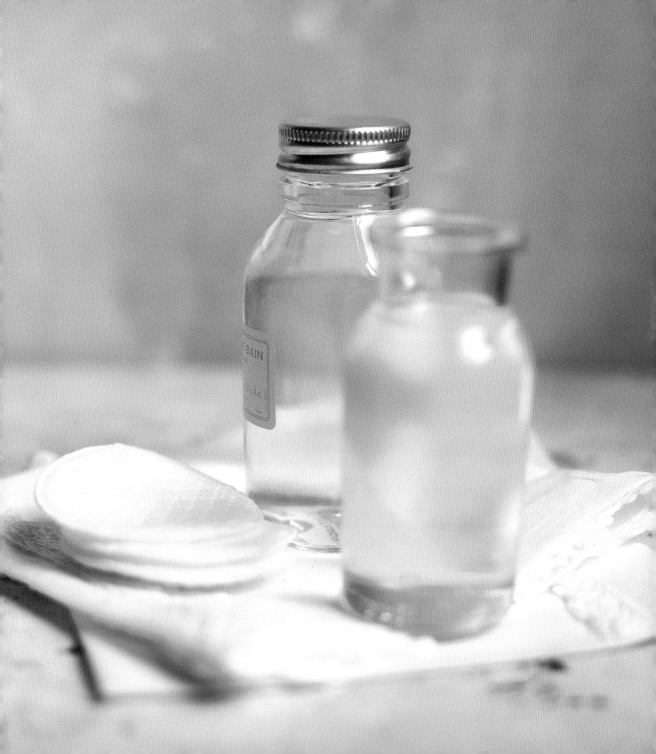

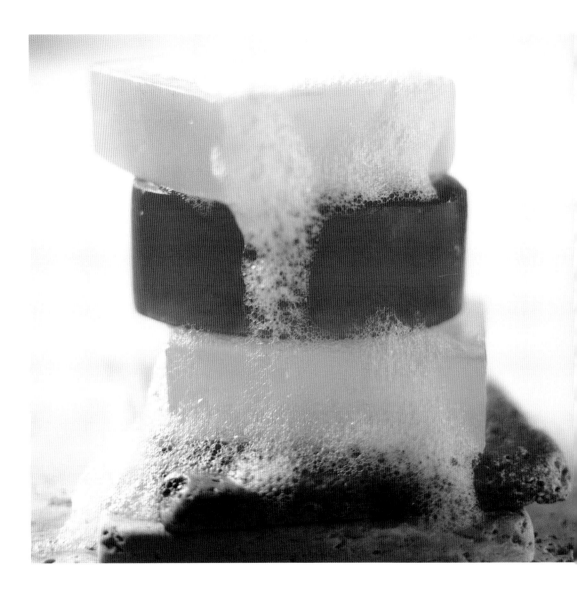

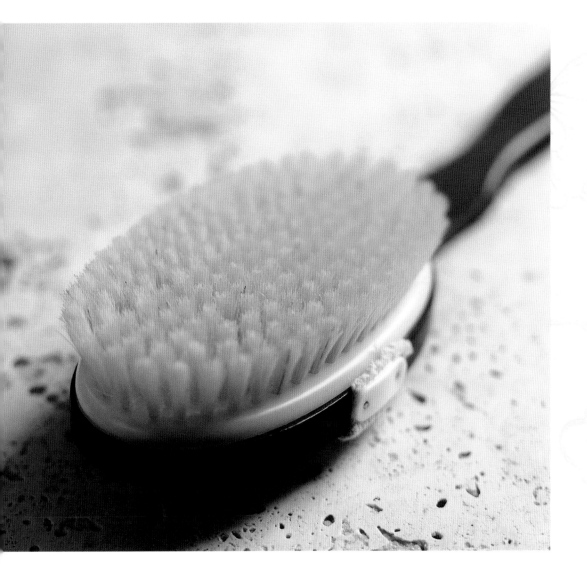

body care

exfoliation

Normal skin sheds old cells and renews them every 28 days. However, this process slows as you age. Exfoliating your skin will help restore it's healthy glow

dry-brush massaging

all skin types

A dry-brush massage is a terrific treatment for skin, as it stimulates circulation and gets rid of the dead cells that can make skin look dull. Use the brush before a bath or shower and brush in a circular movement all over your body, paying special attention to areas where there are glands, such as the armpits, groin and just below the collarbone. Be gentle on breasts and around the genital area.

body scrub

all skin types

This scrub will thoroughly cleanse the skin. You can use either salt or sugar — try both to see which you prefer. The salt and sugar act as exfoliants and the oil moisturizes, so your skin is left feeling silky smooth.

Combine 4–5 teaspoons sugar or salt with 1 teaspoon light olive oil and 1 drop essential oil of your choice and mix well. To use, wet your whole body in the shower, then turn the water off. Apply the sugar or salt scrub and massage it into your skin. Don't use it on your face until you are sure that it's not too abrasive. Rinse well.

Inexpensive, long-handled brushes can be purchased at pharmacies and variety stores.

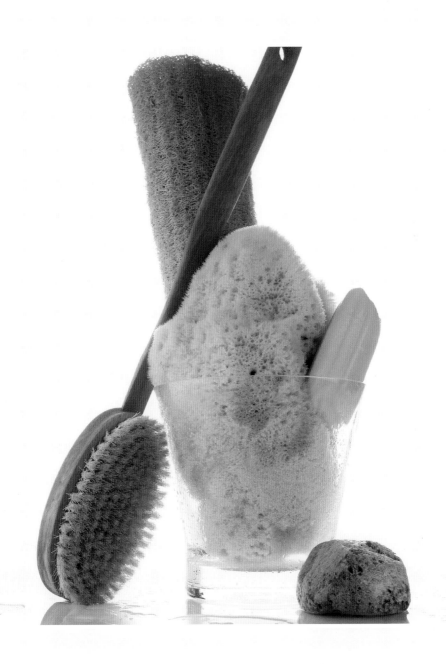

tamarind body polisher

all skin types

Tamarind is a whitening fruit high in alpha hydroxy acids (AHAs) and is a great agent to exfoliate the skin.

ingredients

2 tablespoons tamarind powder

2 tablespoons rice flour

2 tablespoons honey

3 drops mandarin essential oil

3 drops juniper essential oil

soya milk

method

Mix all the ingredients together with enough soya milk to form a paste.

To use, massage your body thoroughly with the mixture, then rinse off.

ginger and sea salt scrub

all skin types

Ginger has a warming effect on the body and is wonderful for aches and pains.

ingredients

20 g (3/4 oz) raw (demerara) sugar

80 g (23/4 oz) fine sea salt

40 ml (11/4 fl oz) apricot kernel oil

25 drops ginger essential oil

method

Mix all the ingredients together. Use a small handful to exfoliate body. This preparation can be used in the bath.

fresh coconut and rice scrub

all skin types, particularly dry and scaly skin

ingredients

60 g (21/4 oz/1 cup) freshly grated coconut

3 tablespoons ground rice

60 ml (2 fl oz/1/4 cup) coconut milk

4 drops of neroli essential oil (or lavender essential oil)

method

Mix the grated coconut with the ground rice and coconut milk. Add the essential oils and mix thoroughly. Scrub your entire body. This recipe can be left on for 15 minutes if your skin is dry. Shower, then moisturize.

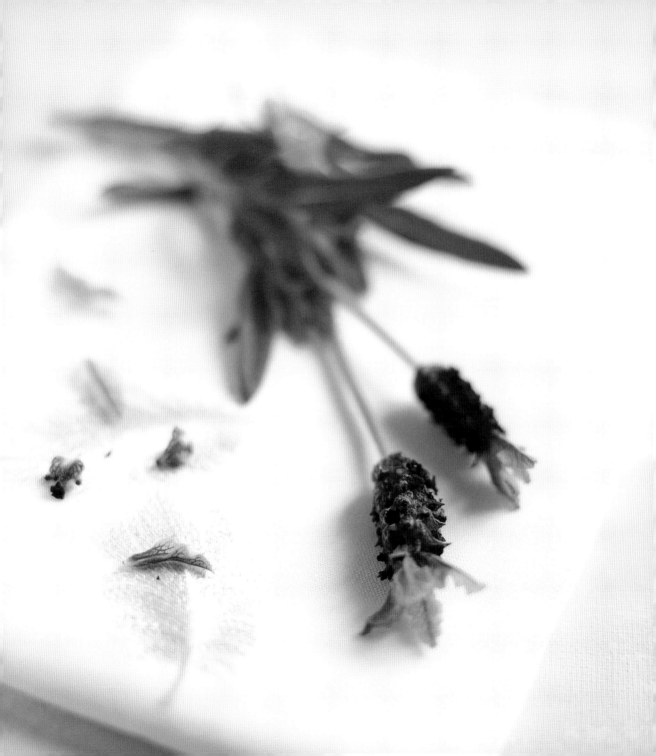

body moisturizers

moisture blocks

all skin types, particularly very dry skin

ingredients

80 g (2³/4 oz) cocoa butter

1 teaspoon coconut oil

1 teaspoon avocado oil

1 teaspoon sweet almond oil

1 teaspoon light olive oil

1 teaspoon jojoba oil

1000 IU vitamin E d'alpha tocopherol

10 drops lavender essential oil

5 drops patchouli essential oil (or sandalwood essential oil)

method

Melt the cocoa butter in the top half of a double boiler. When melted, remove from the heat and add all the remaining ingredients, except for the essential oils (prick the vitamin capsules and squeeze out the contents).

Cool the mixture slightly, then add the essential oils and mix thoroughly. Pour into little chocolate moulds or mini muffin tins. Place in the refrigerator to cool. Moisture blocks can be used on the body after showering, while the skin is still slightly damp.

aloe vera body moisture

all skin types

ingredients

20 g ($3/4$ oz) cocoa butter

5 g ($1/8$ oz) beeswax

10 g ($1/4$ oz) vegetable glycerine

120 g ($41/4$ oz) aloe vera gel

20 ml ($1/2$ fl oz) apricot kernel oil (or sweet almond oil)

2 teaspoons jojoba oil

1 teaspoon vitamin E oil

10 drops lavender essential oil

10 drops geranium essential oil

10 drops palmarosa essential oil

method

Heat the cocoa butter and beeswax in the top half of a double boiler stirring constantly. At the same time, warm the vegetable glycerine and aloe vera gel in a saucepan.

Take both mixtures off the stove and slowly pour the aloe vera mixture into the beeswax mixture and stir until cool. Add the apricot kernel, jojoba and vitamin E oils, and essential oils and mix well.

rich body butter

dry/undernourished skin, also good for psoriasis and eczema

ingredients

100 g (3$^{1}/_{2}$ oz) cocoa butter

10 g ($^{1}/_{4}$ oz) beeswax

55 ml (1$^{3}/_{4}$ fl oz) coconut oil

20 ml ($^{1}/_{2}$ fl oz) jojoba oil

30 ml (1 fl oz) sweet almond oil

20 ml ($^{1}/_{2}$ fl oz) avocado oil

$^{1}/_{2}$ teaspoon vitamin E oil (as preservative)

1 teaspoon vegetable glycerine

50 drops essential oil of your choice

method

Gently melt the cocoa butter and beeswax in the top half of a double boiler. Remove from the heat and add the coconut, jojoba, sweet almond, avocado and vitamin E oils and stir through.

Leave to cool for 10–15 minutes, then add the vegetable glycerine and essential oil. Stir thoroughly. Spoon into glass containers and store in a cool, dry place.

body butter

all skin types, particularly dry, scaly skin

ingredients

1 teaspoon finely grated, tightly packed beeswax

4 teaspoons cocoa butter

1 teaspoon coconut oil

1 teaspoon shea butter, chopped

2 teaspoons cold-pressed avocado oil

40 ml (1¼ fl oz) sweet almond oil

1000 IU vitamin E d'alpha tocopherol

4 drops ylang-ylang essential oil

2 drops sandalwood essential oil

method

Heat the beeswax and cocoa butter in the top half of a double boiler until melted. Remove from the heat and add the coconut oil, stirring until it has melted. Cool, until the outside of the container feels just a little hotter than your hand.

Add the shea butter, avocado and sweet almond oils, beating with a whisk until smooth. Prick the vitamin capsules and squeeze the contents into the mixture. Add the essential oils, a drop at a time, beating after each addition until thoroughly blended. Spoon into sterilized jars.

Avocado is very nourishing for dry or dehydrated skin.

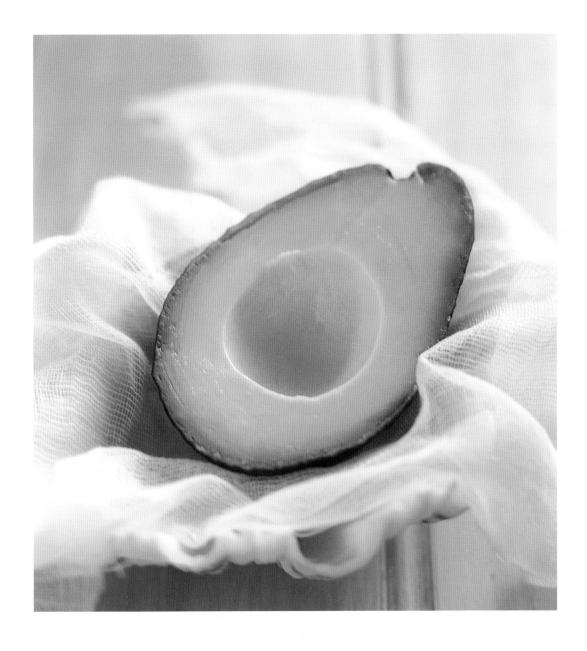

body nourisher

all skin types

ingredients

1 tablespoon cocoa butter

1 teaspoon beeswax

1 tablespoon shea butter, grated

1 teaspoon wheat germ oil

1 teaspoon avocado oil

40 ml (1 1/4 fl oz) apricot kernel oil

1/4 teaspoon vitamin E oil

5 drops palmarosa essential oil

5 drops sandalwood essential oil

method

Heat the cocoa butter and beeswax in the top half of a double boiler until melted. Remove from the heat. Add the shea butter and wheat germ, avocado, apricot kernel and vitamin E oils and beat until smooth. Add the essential oils and mix thoroughly. Spoon into sterilized containers.

cellulite and fluid retention body oil

all skin types

ingredients

20 drops juniper essential oil

10 drops mandarin essential oil

20 drops grapefruit essential oil (or lemon essential oil)

55 ml (1 3/4 fl oz) apricot kernel oil

55 ml (1 3/4 fl oz) macadamia nut oil (or camellia oil)

method

Add the essential oils to the apricot kernel and macadamia nut oils and leave to synergize for 2–3 days. Massage over your entire body twice a day. Rub clockwise on your abdomen.

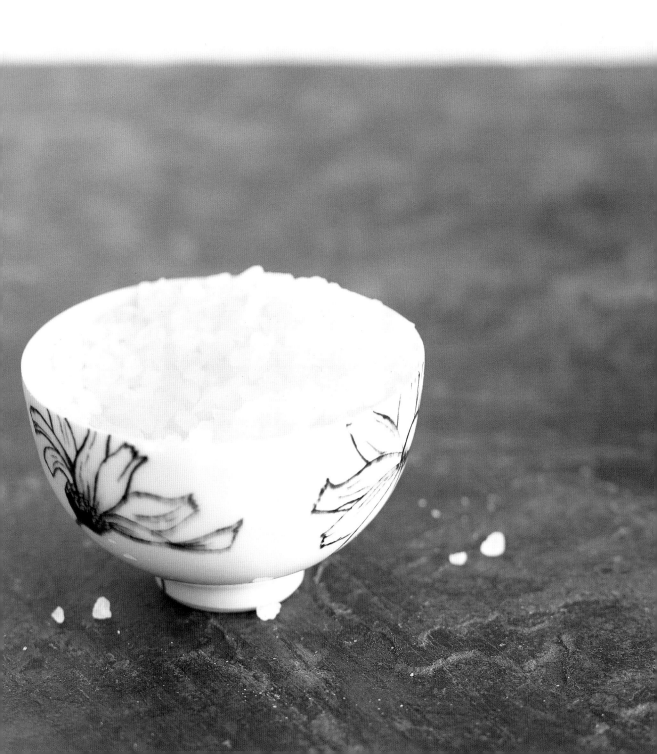

body treatments

papaya and kiwi body mask

all skin types

ingredients

3 tablespoons salt

250 g (9 oz/1 cup) plain yoghurt

1 teaspoon honey

70 g (2 1/2 oz/1 cup) mashed papaya

70 g (2 1/2 oz/1 cup) mashed kiwi fruit

2 teaspoons apricot kernel oil

method

Mix the salt with the yoghurt, then combine with the remaining ingredients. Scrub your body with the mixture. Leave on as a mask for 15-20 minutes, then rinse off. Apply Rich Body Butter (see page 109).

nourishing body oil treatment

all skin types

ingredients

for dry skin

2 teaspoons jojoba oil

2 teaspoons wheat germ oil

2 teaspoons apricot kernel oil

20 ml ($1/2$ fl oz) macadamia nut oil

10 drops palmarosa essential oil

8 drops geranium essential oil (or 4 drops
   ylang-ylang essential oil)

for other skin types

20 ml ($1/2$ fl oz) jojoba oil

2 teaspoons grapeseed oil

20 ml ($1/2$ fl oz) apricot kernel oil

10 drops lavender essential oil

6 drops lemon essential oil

method

Combine all the ingredients in a 55 ml ($13/4$ fl oz) dark bottle and shake well. Store for 3 days in a cool, dark place to synergize.

To use, apply over body after showering.

spider vein treatment

for legs only

This recipe is designed to treat spider veins, not varicose veins.

ingredients

45 ml (1¹/2 fl oz) sweet almond oil

6 drops cypress essential oil

4 drops lemon essential oil

4 drops juniper essential oil

2 drops geranium essential oil

method

Combine all the ingredients in a dark bottle. Leave to synergize for 2–3 days.

To use, rub lightly into areas, where needed, twice a day.

aromatherapy massage oils

Massage strokes should work in harmony with the body's blood flow — always massage towards the heart.

basic massage oil

all skin types

ingredients

80 ml (2^1/$_2$ fl oz/^{1}/$_3$ cup) fractionated coconut oil

(or macadamia oil)

2 teaspoons sweet almond oil

2 teaspoons avocado oil

1000 IU vitamin E d'alpha tocopherol

method

Mix all ingredients together in a 100 ml (3^1/$_2$ fl oz) bottle (prick the vitamin capsules and squeeze out the contents). Shake well to mix.

Dark bottles protect essential oils and their properties, which are adversely affected by light and heat.

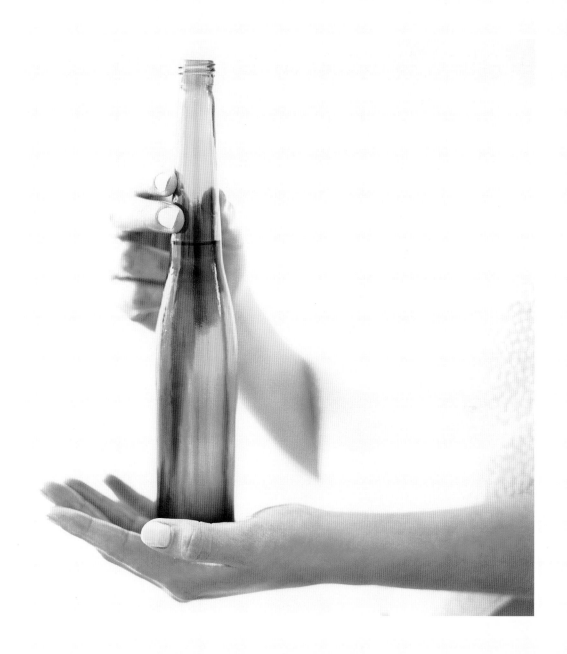

aching bodies

all skin types

This is great for an after-exercise massage, when you ache all over.

ingredients

20 drops lavender essential oil

10 drops rosemary essential oil

10 drops clary sage essential oil

5 drops peppermint essential oil

5 drops cypress essential oil

method

Add the essential oils to an entire bottle of Basic Massage Oil (see page 118). Shake well to mix.

sleep aid

all skin types

This blend will ensure a good night's sleep. Do not use for more than 3 weeks.

ingredients

10 drops chamomile essential oil

20 drops lavender essential oil

10 drops marjoram essential oil

10 drops sandalwood essential oil

method

Add the essential oils to an entire bottle of Basic Massage Oil (see page 118). Shake well to mix.

stress relief

all skin types

This is a great stress reliever for when you are tired from too much thinking and worrying.

ingredients

10 drops lavender essential oil

20 drops chamomile essential oil

10 drops geranium essential oil

5 drops cedarwood essential oil

5 drops peppermint essential oil

method

Add the essential oils to an entire bottle of Basic Massage Oil (see page 118). Shake well to mix.

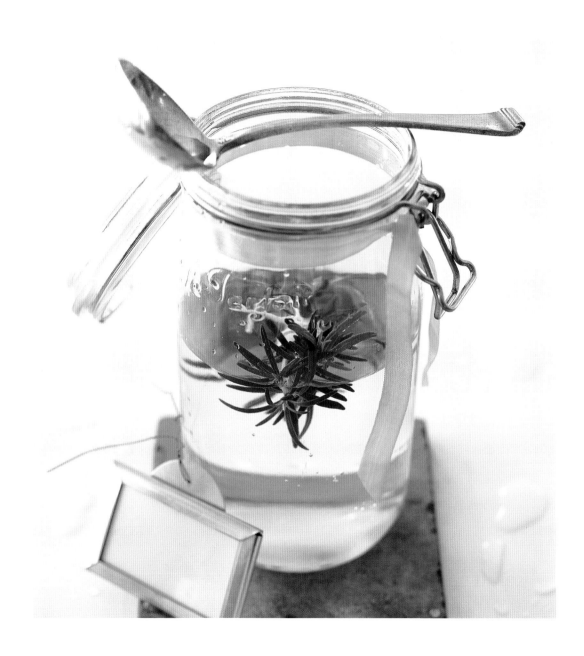

bath mixtures

Always keep the temperature of your bath to 35°C (95°F). Any hotter will raise your pulse rate, leaving you feeling tired.

bath herb 'soup'

all skin types

Fresh herbs in the bath hydrate and soothe the skin but it's not much fun having a bath with twigs and leaves floating around in it. Instead, use the following method.

Put a handful of fresh herbs in a saucepan. Cover the herbs with water, then add 20–40 ml (1/2–1 1/4 fl oz) of cider vinegar. Cover the pan with a lid and simmer over low heat for 20 minutes. Strain (you can add the herbs to your compost bucket) and pour the rich herb soup into the bath or sponge it over your body when you have finished showering. The cider vinegar creates the correct acid balance for your skin and also extracts more properties from the herbs than water alone would do.

herb and oats bath mixture

all skin types

This mixture contains skin–softening oats.

ingredients

55 g (2 oz/2 cups) dried lavender heads

60 g (2^1/$_4$ oz/1 cup) dried rosemary leaves

30 g (1 oz/1 cup) dried peppermint leaves

20 g (^{3}/$_4$ oz/^{1}/$_2$ cup) dried comfrey leaves*

110 g (3^3/$_4$ oz/1 cup) rolled oats

10 drops peppermint essential oil

method

Crumble the dried herbs until the mixture resembles tea leaves. Mix in the oats. Drizzle the essential oil over the herbs and oats, stirring gently. Store the mixture in a tightly sealed jar.

To use, add to your bath 40–90 g (1^1/$_2$–3^1/$_4$ oz/^{1}/$_4$–^{1}/$_2$ cup) of the mixture tied in a muslin bag.

* Comfrey is a restricted substance in some countries.

floral bath mixture

all skin types

ingredients

50 g (1³/4 oz/2 cups) scented dried rose petals

60 g (2¹/4 oz/2 cups) dried rose geranium leaves

10 g (¹/4 oz/¹/2 cup) dried lavender flowers and leaves

15 drops ylang-ylang essential oil (or jasmine essential oil)

method

Crumble the herbs until the mixture resembles tea leaves. Drizzle the essential oil over the herbs, stirring gently. Store the mix in a tightly sealed jar. To use, add to your bath 40–90 g (1¹/2–3¹/4 oz/¹/4–¹/2 cup) of the mixture tied in a muslin bag.

golden bubble bath

normal/oily skin

ingredients

125 ml (4 fl oz/¹/2 cup) golden-coloured shampoo*

1 egg, beaten

1 teaspoon runny honey

1 teaspoon vegetable glycerine

20 drops essential oil of your choice

method

Combine all the ingredients, then bottle. Keep refrigerated and use within 2 weeks. To use, slowly trickle about 60 ml (2 fl oz/¹/4 cup) of the mixture under a fast-running tap to maximize the bubbles.

* Use a good-quality organic shampoo, purchased from a health food store.

citrus refresher bath mixture

all skin types

This sprightly bath blend relieves that frazzled feeling after a hot day.

ingredients

60 g (2^1/$_4$ oz/2 cups) dried lemon grass

10 g (^{1}/$_4$ oz/1 cup) dried lemon verbena leaves

25 g (1 oz/^{1}/$_2$ cup) dried mint leaves

1 tablespoon dried, ground lemon peel

1 tablespoon dried, ground orange peel (or mandarin peel)

10 drops peppermint essential oil

method

Crumble the dried herbs and citrus peel until the mixture resembles tea leaves. Drizzle the essential oil over the mixture, stirring gently. Store in a tightly sealed jar.

To use, add to your bath 40–90 g (1^1/$_2$–3^1/$_4$ oz/^{1}/$_4$–^{1}/$_2$ cup) of the mixture tied in a muslin bag. Run hot water over the mixture, then add cold water until the bath is the correct temperature.

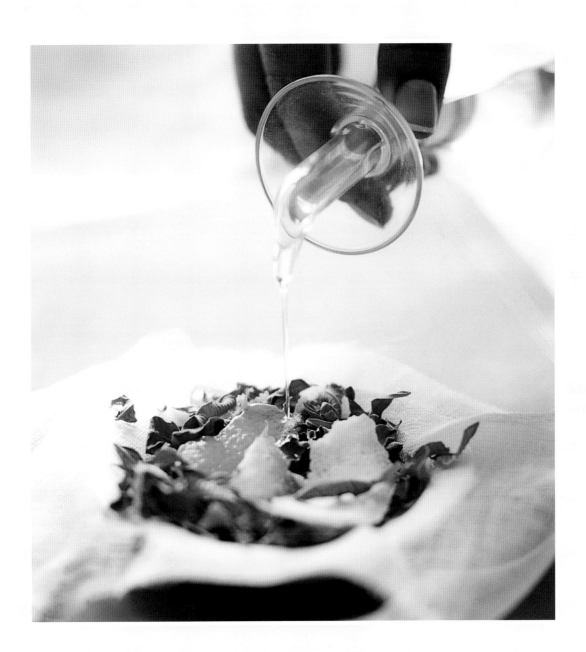

bath oils

Relax and de-stress with these beautiful bath oils.

st clements bath oil

all skin types

ingredients

40 drops lemon essential oil

20 drops orange essential oil

1 drop essential oil of cloves

4 teaspoons tincture of benzoin

125 ml (4 fl oz/^{1}/$_2$ cup) vodka

50 g (1^3/$_4$ oz) anhydrous lanolin

4 teaspoons runny honey

375 ml (13 fl oz/1^1/$_2$ cups) herb oil base

method

Dissolve the essential oils and tincture in the vodka.

Heat the lanolin and honey in the top half of a double boiler, taking care not to overheat. Remove from the heat and cool to 45°C (113°F).

Slowly stir the vodka and oil blend into the lanolin and honey mixture, then bottle. Add about 60 ml (2 fl oz/^{1}/$_4$ cup) to the bath as the water is running.

intensive treatment bath oil

all skin types

ingredients

125 ml (4 fl oz/1/2 cup) brandy (or vodka)

10 drops petitgrain essential oil

10 drops bergamot essential oil

10 drops rosemary essential oil

10 drops lemon essential oil

10 drops patchouli essential oil

2 teaspoons vegetable glycerine

2 teaspoons sweet almond oil (or macadamia oil)

method

Put all the ingredients in a bottle. Shake well and leave for 3 days to blend.

Pour *1 teaspoon of the oil only* on the surface of the bath just before you step in. A potent oil!

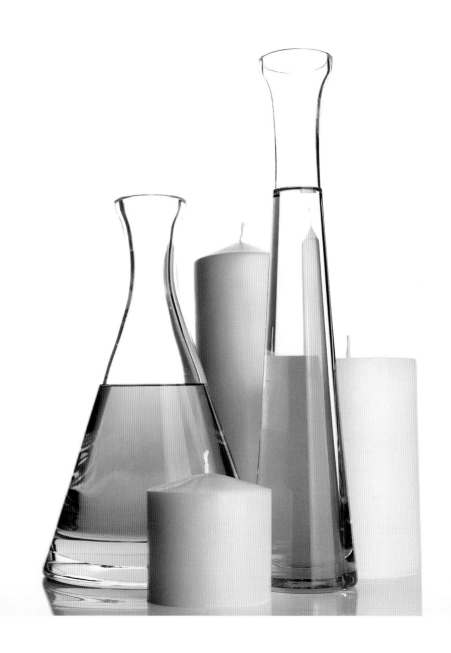

lavender bath oil

all skin types

This oil will relieve dry, itchy skin and relax tired muscles.

ingredients

1 egg

2 teaspoons cider vinegar

40 ml (1 1/4 fl oz) vodka

2 teaspoons vegetable glycerine

125 ml (4 fl oz/1/2 cup) light olive oil (or macadamia oil)

20 drops lavender essential oil

10 drops patchouli essential oil

5 drops rosemary essential oil

1 tablespoon homemade shampoo (see pages 167 or 168)

method

Beat the egg, cider vinegar, vodka, glycerine, olive oil and essential oils together. Stir in the shampoo, mix well, then bottle. Keep refrigerated and use within 2 weeks.

To use, add about 60 ml (2 fl oz/1/4 cup) of the mixture to the bath, as the water is running.

aromatherapy bath oils

The following blends are sufficient for one bath. To avoid floating 'hot spots' of unmixed essential oil, it is best to mix the essential oils with 20 ml ($1/2$ fl oz) of either full-cream (whole) milk or sweet almond oil before adding them to the bath.

ingredients

skin deodorizing blend

4 drops clary sage essential oil

2 drops eucalyptus essential oil

2 drops tea tree essential oil

2 drops peppermint essential oil

dry skin blend

4 drops chamomile essential oil

4 drops geranium essential oil

2 drops patchouli essential oil

oily skin blend

5 drops lemon essential oil

3 drops ylang-ylang essential oil

2 drops cypress essential oil

spotty skin blend

2 drops eucalyptus essential oil

2 drops thyme essential oil

4 drops lavender essential oil

2 drops chamomile essential oil

aromatic blend

1 drop lavender essential oil

2 drops grapefruit essential oil

2 drops geranium essential oil

2 drops ylang-ylang essential oil

2 drops patchouli essential oil

relaxing blend

4 drops chamomile essential oil

3 drops lavender essential oil

3 drops ylang-ylang essential oil

bath salts

To use the following bath salts, mix all the dry ingredients together. Add the essential oils, drop by drop, stirring constantly to prevent caking. Put the mixture in a jar and shake daily for a few days to blend the ingredients. To use, sprinkle about 30–60 g (1–2^1/$_4$ oz/^{1}/$_4$–^{1}/$_2$ cup) of the mixture in the bath, as it is running.

sandalwood salts

ingredients

100 g (3^1/$_2$ oz/^{1}/$_2$ cup) tartaric acid

125 g (4^1/$_2$ oz/^{1}/$_2$ cup) bicarbonate of soda (baking soda)

30 g (1 oz/^{1}/$_4$ cup) cornflour (cornstarch)

20 drops geranium essential oil

2 drops grapefruit essential oil

4 drops sandalwood essential oil

scent of the forest salts

ingredients

125 g (4^1/$_2$ oz/^{1}/$_2$ cup) bicarbonate of soda (baking soda)

140 g (5 oz/^{1}/$_2$ cup) Epsom salts

100 g (3^1/$_2$ oz/^{1}/$_2$ cup) tartaric acid

140 g (5 oz/1 cup) Irish moss, ground to a powder

850 g (1 lb 14 oz/3 cups) fine sea salt

4 drops pine essential oil

20 drops eucalyptus essential oil

It is better to use natural materials in your bathroom, such as cotton, for towels, face cloths and bathmats.

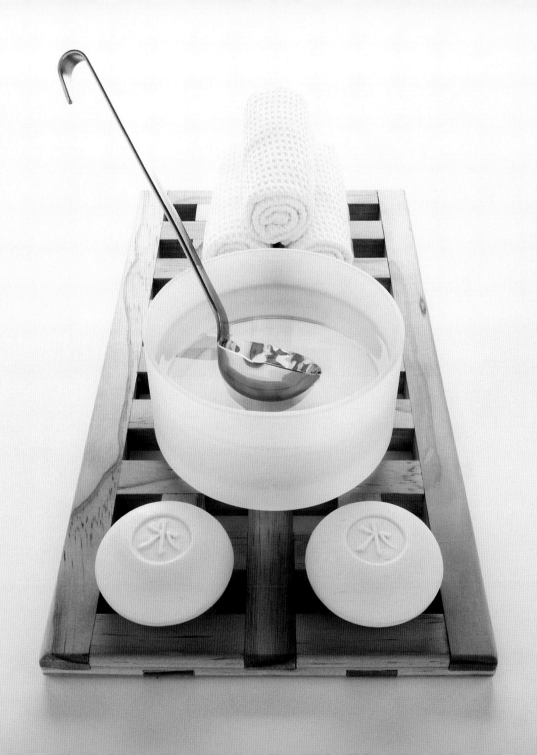

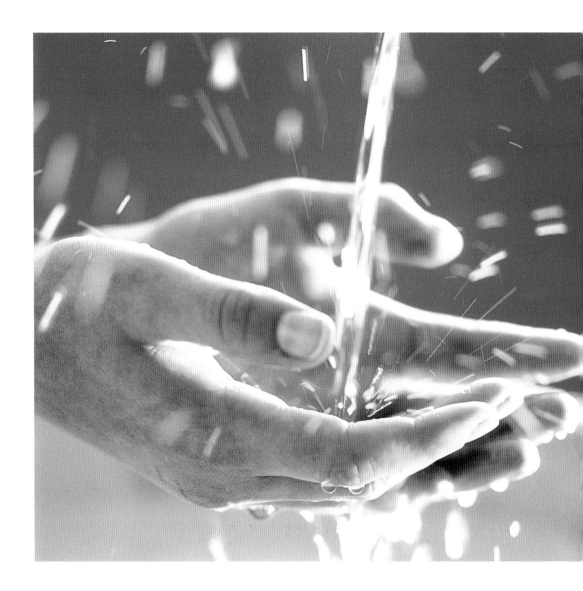

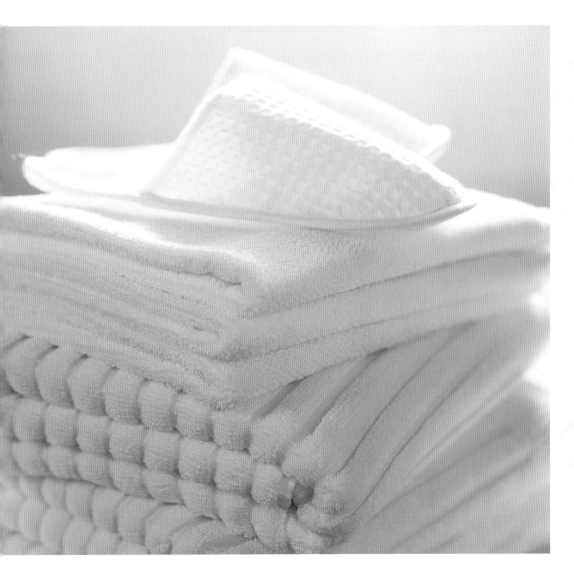

hand and foot care

hand cleansers

gentle hand cleanser

all skin types

This simple hand cleanser is thorough but gentle.

ingredients

50 g (1^3/$_4$ oz) finely powdered soap

50 g (1^3/$_4$ oz) fine sawdust

^{1}/$_2$ teaspoon borax*

method

Mix all the ingredients together. Store in an airtight jar.

To use, put a teaspoonful of the mixture on the palm of your hand, drizzle on enough water to form a paste and work this up to a lather. Rinse your hands and pat them dry.

*   Recipes containing borax should not be used for infants and children, pregnant women or those with sensitive skin.

coconut and lemon hand cleanser

all skin types

ingredients

1 tablespoon grated coconut

1 teaspoon coconut oil

juice of 1/4 lemon

method

Combine all the ingredients. Rub the mixture into your hands, then rinse with warm water. Follow with moisturizer.

olive oil de-greaser

all skin types

ingredients

20 ml (1/2 fl oz) olive oil

juice of 1/2 lemon

method

Mix the olive oil and lemon juice together. Rub the mixture into your hands, then wash off with warm water.

quick lemon and sugar scrub

all skin types

This scrub will leave your hands feeling like smooth satin.

ingredients

20 ml ($1/2$ fl oz) lemon juice

1–2 tablespoons sugar

method

Mix together the lemon juice and sugar and use the scrub immediately.

To use, massage the mixture into your hands, then rinse off and dry. Apply a little of the Lemon and Almond Hand Cream (see page 143).

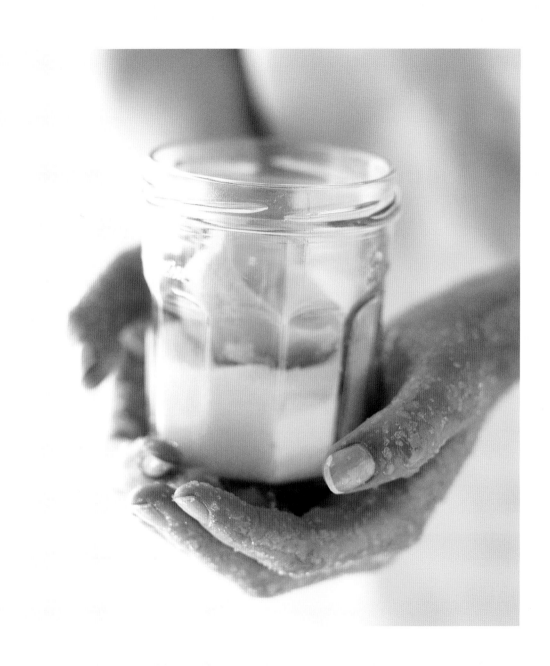

hand moisturizers

Sweet almond oil is a great treatment for dry and chafed skin, while glycerine will prevent moisture evaporation. Essential oils are also particularly good for hands and nails as they work very quickly and are readily absorbed into the skin without leaving an unpleasant greasy feeling.

rosewater and glycerine hand lotion

all skin types

The vinegar in this recipe restores the acid balance of the skin and helps the other ingredients to be easily absorbed into the skin.

ingredients

20 ml ($1/2$ fl oz) rosewater

2 teaspoons vegetable glycerine

$1/2$ teaspoon white wine vinegar

$1/2$ teaspoon runny honey

10 drops lemon essential oil

method

Mix all the ingredients together in a 55 ml ($13/4$ fl oz) bottle. Shake well.

lemon and almond hand cream

dry skin

ingredients

Phase A

30 ml (1 fl oz) vegetable glycerine

20 ml ($1/2$ fl oz) distilled water

1 teaspoon borax*

Phase B

20 g ($3/4$ oz) grated beeswax

60 ml (2 fl oz/$1/4$ cup) sweet almond oil

1 teaspoon castor oil

60 ml (2 fl oz/$1/4$ cup) olive oil

Phase C

20 drops lemon essential oil

20 drops lavender essential oil

method

Gently heat all Phase A ingredients until the borax is dissolved. Melt the Phase B ingredients gently in the top half of a double boiler until the mixture is liquid but not overheated.

Slowly trickle the Phase A mixture into the Phase B mixture. Stir constantly and reheat slightly if the mixture begins to solidify. Add the Phase C essential oils when the outside of the container feels a little hotter than your hand and the mixture is still liquid. Stir until the essential oils are completely incorporated. Pour into sterilized containers and cap at once.

*   Recipes containing borax should not be used for infants and children, pregnant women or those with sensitive skin.

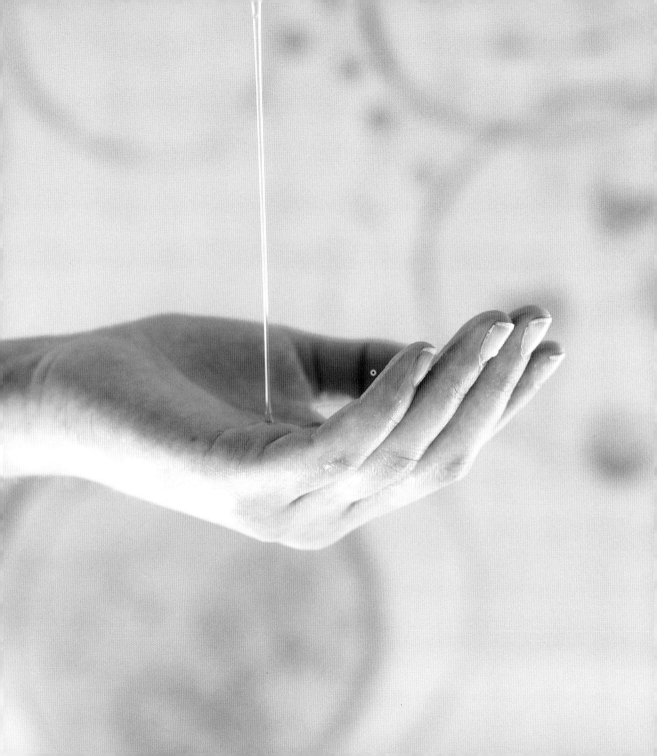

honey hand lotion

all skin types

This simple hand lotion is easy to make and use. It will separate on standing, so it should be shaken before use.

ingredients

    1 tablespoon runny honey
    1 teaspoon avocado oil
    1 teaspoon sweet almond oil
    80 ml (2¹/₂ fl oz/¹/₃ cup) rosewater
    1 teaspoon vegetable glycerine
    1 tablespoon white wine vinegar

method

Gently heat the honey and oils in a saucepan until the honey is melted. Heat the rosewater, glycerine and vinegar in another saucepan until they are roughly the same temperature as the oils and honey.

Add the rosewater mixture to the oil and honey mixture and beat together until cool. Bottle and shake well.

silky hand cream

dry skin

ingredients

1$^1/_2$ teaspoons cocoa butter

1 teaspoon almond oil

$^1/_2$ teaspoon beeswax

60 ml (2 fl oz/$^1/_4$ cup) distilled water (or rosewater)

$^1/_2$ teaspoon borax*

20 drops essential oil of your choice

method

Melt the cocoa butter, almond oil and beeswax in the top half of a double boiler. In a separate saucepan heat the distilled water slightly and stir in the borax until dissolved. Pour the oil and beeswax blend into the water and mix slowly until the mixture reaches a creamy consistency. Stir until the cream cools. Add the essential oils and mix thoroughly. Spoon into glass containers.

nail hardener

all skin types

ingredients

1 teaspoon apple cider vinegar

juice of $^1/_4$ lemon

10 drops lemon essential oil

method

Combine all the ingredients. Paint onto your nails daily. In 4–6 weeks you should see an improvement to your nails.

*   Recipes containing borax should not be used for infants and children, pregnant women or those with sensitive skin.

nourishing nail conditioner

all skin types

ingredients

30 ml (1 fl oz) sweet almond oil

2 teaspoons macadamia nut oil

15 drops lemon essential oil

4 drops sandalwood essential oil

1/4 teaspoon vitamin E oil

method

Combine all the ingredients and store in a dark bottle. Rub into your nails and hands twice a day.

hand and nail buffer

all skin types

This nourishing hand cream can also be used as a hand mask.

ingredients

5 g (1/8 oz) beeswax, grated

5 g (1/8 oz) cocoa butter

10 g (1/4 oz) lanolin

20 ml (1/2 fl oz) jojoba oil

20 drops essential oils of your choice

method

Melt the beeswax and cocoa butter in the top half of a double boiler. Add the lanolin and jojoba oil and stir until all the ingredients are heated. Allow to cool slightly, then add the essential oils and stir well. Apply to hands, leave on for 15–20 minutes, then rinse off.

hand and nail essential oil

all skin types

ingredients

45 ml (1$^1/_2$ fl oz) macadamia oil

1 teaspoon avocado oil

1 teaspoon carrot seed oil

1$^1/_2$ teaspoons jojoba oil

2 teaspoons evening primrose oil

15 drops lemon essential oil

10 drops rosemary essential oil

10 drops geranium essential oil

5 drops patchouli essential oil

1000 IU vitamin E d'alpha tocopherol

method

Mix all the ingredients in a 55 ml (1$^3/_4$ fl oz) bottle (prick the vitamin capsules and squeeze out the contents). Shake well to mix, then leave for 4 days to blend. Store in a cool dark place. To use, shake the bottle and then massage 4–5 drops into your hands and around the nail bed.

honey balm

all skin types

Melt 1 teaspoon beeswax with $^1/_2$ teaspoon olive oil. Allow to cool slightly, then add 1 teaspoon honey and 2 drops lavender essential oil and mix well. Apply the cream all over your hands when needed.

Hands are exposed to harsh and drying household cleaning products. Repair them with an intensive essential oil treatment.

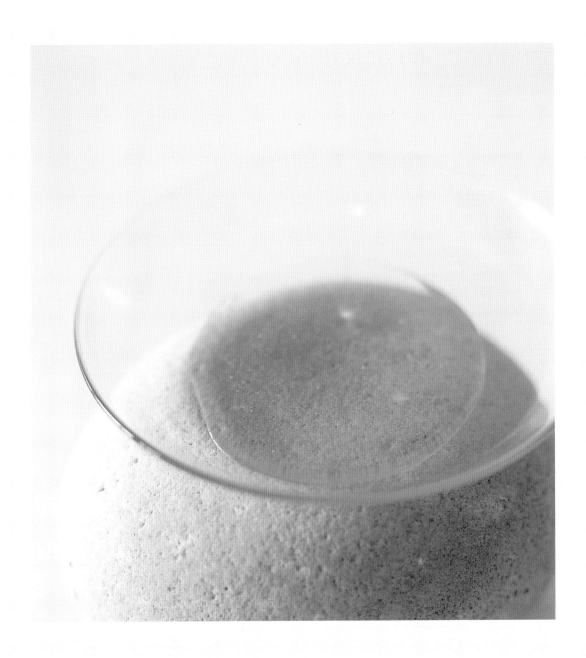

foot cleansers

To massage your feet, apply your chosen oil and knead the sole of each foot. Then slowly work over the top of each foot and up the leg with a long, sweeping action.

herbal foot bath

all skin types

To make this soothing bath for sore feet, first brew a strong tea of finely chopped fresh herbs to half fill a bowl large enough for both feet. Use as many of the following herbs as possible: lavender, sage, pine needles, pennyroyal, rosemary and yarrow.

Have the herbal water as hot as you can bear. Soak your feet for 10–15 minutes. Finish by plunging your feet into a bowl of cold water mixed with 80 ml (2$\frac{1}{2}$ fl oz/$\frac{1}{3}$ cup) witch hazel. Pat your feet dry and massage with Aromatherapy Foot Oil (see opposite page).

aromatherapy foot oil

all skin types

Your feet will thank you for massaging them with this beautiful oil. Not only does it ease the pain of tired feet but it also soothes the irritating symptoms of tinea.

ingredients

20 ml ($1/2$ fl oz) vodka

45 ml ($1^1/2$ fl oz) light olive oil

2 teaspoons avocado oil

2 teaspoons jojoba oil

2 teaspoons sweet almond oil

20 drops peppermint essential oil

10 drops tea tree essential oil

30 drops lavender essential oil

20 drops cypress essential oil

method

Put all the ingredients into a 100 ml ($3^1/2$ fl oz) bottle. Shake well for several minutes. Leave for 4 days to blend. Store in a cool dark place.

To use, first wash or soak your feet, then dry them thoroughly. Shake the bottle well and massage a little of the oil into your feet until it is absorbed.

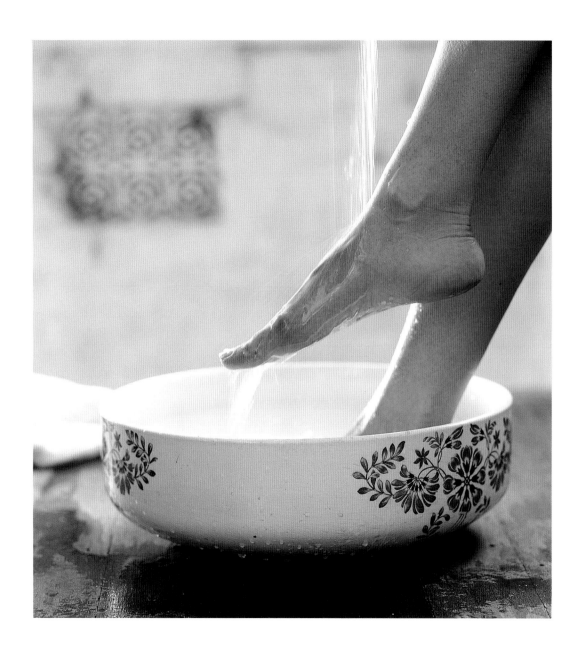

beach polish

all skin types

ingredients

2 tablespoons fine sea salt

45 g (1^1/$_2$ oz) beach sand

100 ml (3^1/$_2$ fl oz) coconut oil

3 drops peppermint essential oil

1 drop tea tree essential oil

method

Combine all the ingredients. Wet your feet and rub the mixture thoroughly over each foot, taking particular care on extra dry areas. Wash off and soak your feet in Floral Foot Fantasy (see below).

floral foot fantasy

all skin types

ingredients

1 pot freshly brewed peppermint tea, strained

1 cup flowers (such as rose petals or chamomile)
    soaked in distilled water, drained

juice of 1 lemon

3 drops lavender essential oil

1 drop peppermint essential oil

method

Scrub feet first with Beach Polish (see above). Combine all the ingredients. Soak feet in the mixture for 10–15 minutes, then rinse and dry. Moisturize thoroughly.

foot powder

all skin types

This powder may be sprinkled inside socks and shoes if you suffer from sweaty feet.

ingredients

100 g ($3^1/2$ oz/1 cup) kaolin powder

60 g ($2^1/4$ oz/$^1/2$ cup) cornflour (cornstarch)

55 g (2 oz/$^1/2$ cup) arrowroot

2 tablespoons powdered dried sage leaves

2 tablespoons powdered dried rosemary

10 drops lavender essential oil

10 drops tea tree essential oil

10 drops tincture of myrrh

10 drops tincture of benzoin

method

Mix all the dry ingredients together, and blend or rub until very fine. Push through a fine sieve. Mix the oils and tinctures together and drip slowly onto the mixed powders, stirring constantly to avoid clumping. Store in a container with a very tight-fitting lid.

foot odour powder

all skin types

ingredients

3 tablespoons bicarbonate of soda (baking soda)

2 drops lemon grass essential oil

2 drops sage essential oil

method

Combine all the ingredients and mix thoroughly. Allow the mixture to dry.

Dust feet twice a day. The powder can also be left in shoes overnight.

fresh cream treat

all skin types

ingredients

40 ml (1^{1}/4 fl oz) pouring (whipping) cream

1 teaspoon olive oil

1 tablespoon aloe vera gel (optional)

10 drops essential oil of your choice

method

Combine all the ingredients. Rub generously into your feet.

Slip your feet into socks and leave on overnight, or for as long as possible.

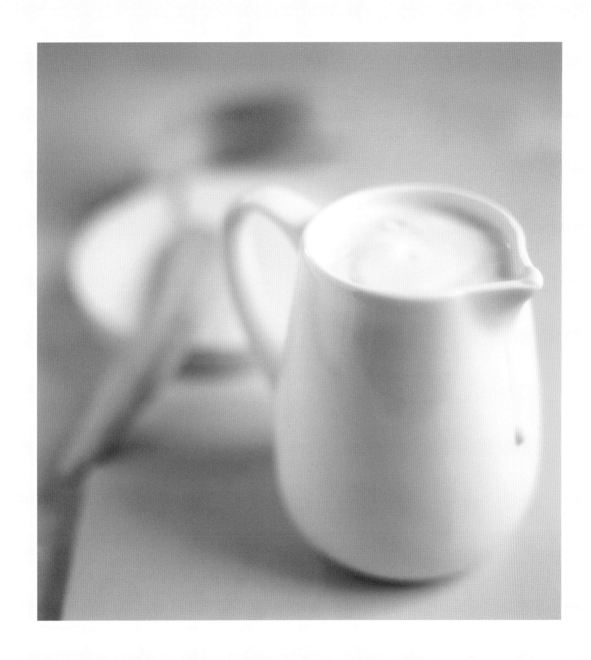

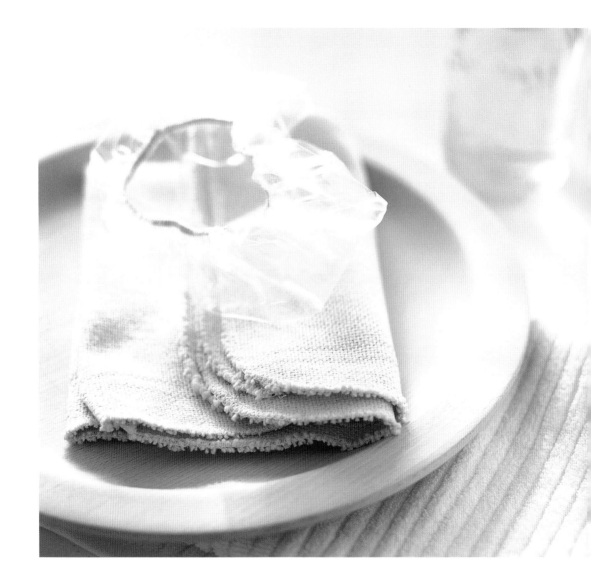

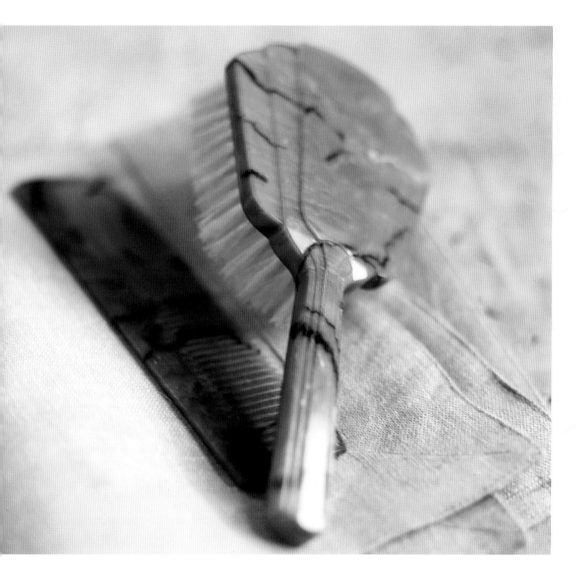

hair care

pre-shampoo treatments

The condition of your hair reflects your inner health. The way to strong, shiny hair is through a nutritious, balanced diet and an effective health and fitness regime.

simple egg treatment

all hair types

This is a really effective protein treatment for hair. Beat two eggs in a bowl until light and frothy. Massage this mixture thoroughly into your hair. Rinse with lukewarm water. If you rinse with hot water you'll end up with scrambled egg in your hair!

hair mayonnaise

all except very oily hair

ingredients

1 egg yolk

3 teaspoons apple cider vinegar

20 ml ($1/2$ fl oz) castor oil

20 ml ($1/2$ fl oz) light olive oil

4 drops lavender essential oil

method

Beat the egg and vinegar together with a wire whisk, or in a blender. Mix the oils together and add to the egg and vinegar mixture in a thin stream until the mixture is thick. Use immediately.

To use, massage the mayonnaise into your hair, cover your hair with a plastic shower cap, then wrap a hot towel around your head. Leave for 20 minutes, then wash your hair using a mild herbal shampoo.

thai fruit tonic

dry/normal/oily hair

ingredients

100 ml (3^1/$_2$ fl oz) coconut oil

130 g (4^1/$_2$ oz) aloe vera gel

6 drops jasmine essential oil (for dry hair)

or

6 drops ylang-ylang essential oil (for normal to oily hair)

method

Combine the coconut oil and aloe vera gel and mix thoroughly. Add the essential oil appropriate for your hair type and blend.

Apply the mixture to your hair and massage. Wrap a hot towel around your head for better absorption. Leave on for at least 10 minutes. Shampoo and condition your hair.

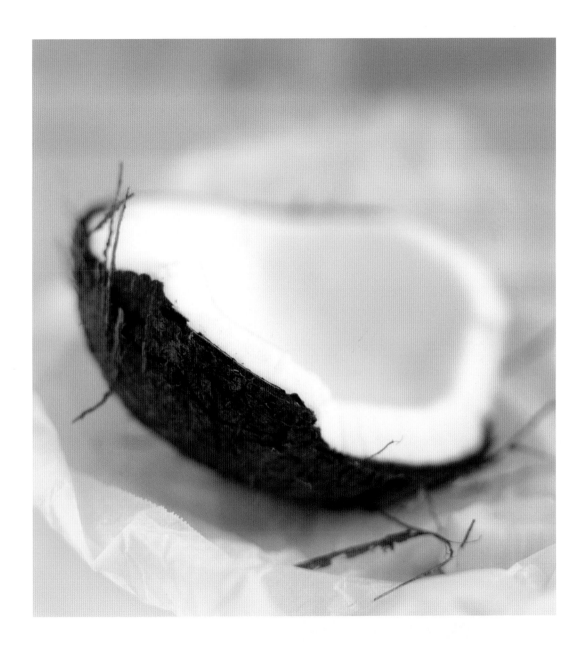

honey and lemon treatment

oily hair

ingredients

1 egg white, beaten

1 teaspoon runny honey

1 teaspoon lemon juice

3 drops lemon essential oil

dried milk powder

method

Combine the egg white, honey, lemon juice and essential oil with 20 ml (^{1}/$_2$ fl oz) water in a small bowl. Add enough milk powder to make a smooth, soft paste. Use immediately.

To use, massage the paste into your hair. Cover your hair with a plastic shower cap, then wrap a hot towel around your head. Leave for 20 minutes, then shampoo your hair with a mild herbal shampoo.

treatment for hair loss

hair loss

ingredients

40 ml (1¼ fl oz) avocado oil

20 ml (½ fl oz) macadamia nut oil (or wheat germ oil)

1 egg

⅛ teaspoon spirulina powder

3 drops rosemary essential oil

2 drops cedarwood essential oil

method

Combine all the ingredients together. Gently massage into your scalp. Put on a shower cap, then wrap a hot towel around your head. Leave for 20–30 minutes. Shampoo directly onto the treatment, then rinse off.

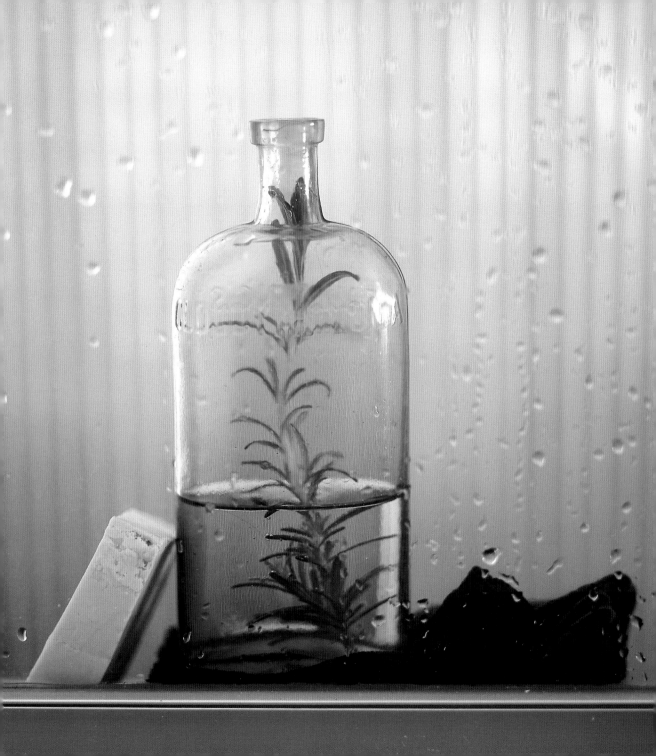

shampoos

simple shampoo

all hair types

ingredients

25 g (1 oz/^{1}/3 cup) tightly packed soap flakes

2 teaspoons borax*

1 litre (35 fl oz/4 cups) very hot distilled water

40 drops lavender essential oil

40 drops rosemary essential oil

20 drops basil essential oil (optional)

method

Dissolve the soap flakes and borax in the hot water. When the mixture has cooled slightly, add the essential oils and stir well to distribute them through the mixture. The mixture may become lumpy on standing, so another good stir will be needed before use.

The shampoo can be poured into a squeezebottle or can simply be scooped out of the mixing jar as you need it. The squeezebottle method is best, as this slippery mixture has a habit of sliding off your hands and hair. Follow with Floral Vinegar Rinse (see page 175).

* Recipes containing borax should not be used for infants and children, pregnant women or those with sensitive skin.

castile shampoo

all hair types

In the following recipe you can use either fresh herbs or essential oils, but remember that a shampoo using fresh herbs won't last as long without preservation as one that uses essential oils.

ingredients

3 tablespoons finely chopped rosemary and lavender

250 ml (9 fl oz/1 cup) distilled water

185 ml (6 fl oz/3/4 cup) liquid Castile soap

or

20 drops lavender essential oil

10 drops rosemary essential oil

185 ml (6 fl oz/3/4 cup) liquid Castile soap

method

To make the herbal option, simmer the herbs and water in a covered saucepan for 30 minutes. Leave overnight if possible. Strain, pour back into the pan and simmer, covered, until reduced to 60 ml (2 fl oz/1/4 cup). Strain through coffee filter paper, add to the Castile soap, mix and then bottle. Follow with Floral Vinegar Rinse (see page 175).

To make the essential oil option, add the essential oils to the Castile soap and mix well. Invert the bottle a couple of times before use. Follow with Floral Vinegar Rinse (see page 175).

protein body shampoo

dry hair

ingredients

250 ml (9 fl oz/1 cup) liquid Castile soap

3 horsetail chestnut extract capsules

1/4 teaspoon vitamin E oil

10 drops lavender essential oil

10 drops rosemary essential oil

method

Combine 55 ml (1³/4 fl oz) of the liquid Castile soap with the contents of the horsetail chestnut capsules (prick the capsules and squeeze out the contents) and mix thoroughly. Add the vitamin E oil and essential oils and mix well. Combine the mixture with the remaining liquid Castile soap. Let stand for 24 hours. Shampoo hair and follow with conditioner.

clay shampoo

damaged hair

Make a tea with 1 tablespoon dried chamomile flowers and 125 ml (4 fl oz/1/2 cup) boiling distilled water, then strain. Combine the tea with 100 g (3¹/2 oz) kaolin clay to form a paste, then add 10 drops essential oil (such as chamomile, lavender, rosemary or lemon). Mix thoroughly. Soak your hair all over with the paste and leave for 3 minutes to 1 hour. Rinse off and follow with conditioner.

anti-dandruff shampoo

dandruff-prone hair

ingredients

250 ml (9 fl oz/1 cup) shampoo base (use either the Simple
   Shampoo (page 167) or the Castile Shampoo (page 168)
20 drops rosemary essential oil
20 drops eucalyptus essential oil
20 drops lemon essential oil

method

Mix all the ingredients together. Store in a squeezebottle. To use, invert the bottle a few times
to mix the oils with the shampoo. Shampoo your hair, paying special attention to the scalp
and massage with the pads of your fingers, not the nails. Rinse well and follow with Floral
Vinegar Rinse (page 175).

nourishing shampoo

normal/dry hair

ingredients

1 cup liquid Castile soap
1 tablespoon carrier oil (such as jojoba, macadamia nut, wheat germ)
8 drops essential oil of your choice

method

Pour 125 ml (4 fl oz/$^1/_2$ cup) water into a bottle with a spray nozzle. Add the liquid Castile
soap, carrier oil and essential oil and lightly shake the bottle. There is no need to use
conditioner with this shampoo unless your hair is very dry.

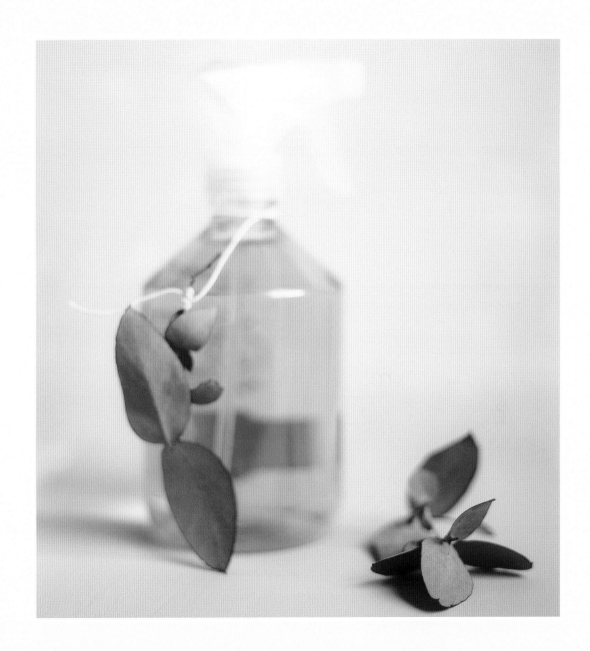

conditioners

lemon conditioner

oily hair

ingredients

40 ml (1^1/$_4$ fl oz) vodka

1 teaspoon runny honey

1 egg white, beaten

2 drops lemon essential oil

1 drop rosemary essential oil

skim milk powder

method

Beat all the ingredients together with enough skim milk powder to form a soft paste.

To use, massage the conditioner into your hair after shampooing. Leave on for a few minutes, then rinse your hair lightly with lukewarm water.

rosemary conditioner

all hair types, except oily

ingredients

1 egg, beaten

1 teaspoon vegetable glycerine

2 drops castor oil

2 drops rosemary essential oil

2 drops lavender essential oil

skim milk powder

method

Beat all the ingredients together with enough skim milk powder to form a soft paste.

To use, massage the conditioner into your hair after shampooing. Leave on for a few minutes, then rinse your hair lightly with lukewarm water.

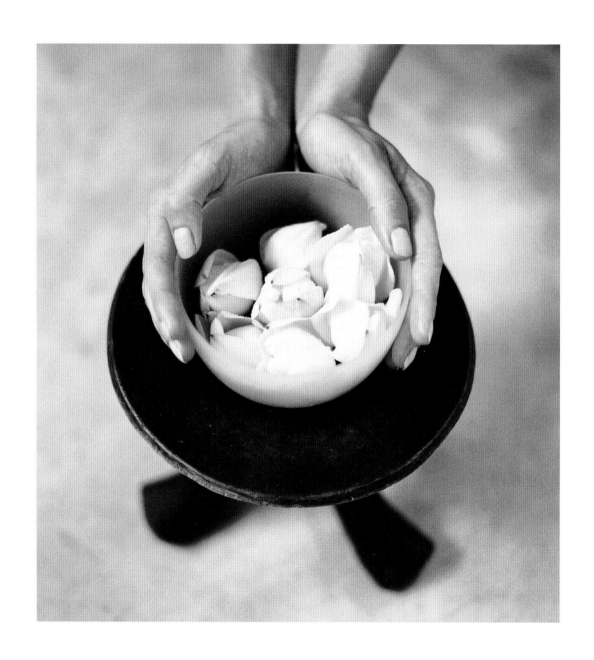

floral vinegar rinse

normal/dry hair

ingredients

40 ml (1^1/4 fl oz) vinegar (white wine or apple cider)

20 drops lavender essential oil

20 drops rosemary essential oil

10 drops geranium essential oil (or lemon essential oil for oily hair)

distilled water

method

Mix the vinegar and essential oils together in a 300 ml (10^1/2 fl oz) bottle with a spray nozzle. Fill to the top with distilled water. Shake well before use. To use, rinse your hair after shampooing, then spray thoroughly with the vinegar rinse. Don't rinse out.

shiny locks

all hair types

ingredients

100 ml (3^1/2 fl oz) distilled water (or floral water)

25 ml (^{3}/4 fl oz) aloe vera juice

25 ml (^{3}/4 fl oz) cucumber juice

25 ml (^{3}/4 fl oz) white wine vinegar

6 drops carrot seed essential oil

8 drops neroli essential oil

method

Combine all the ingredients. Pour over your hair as a final rinse.

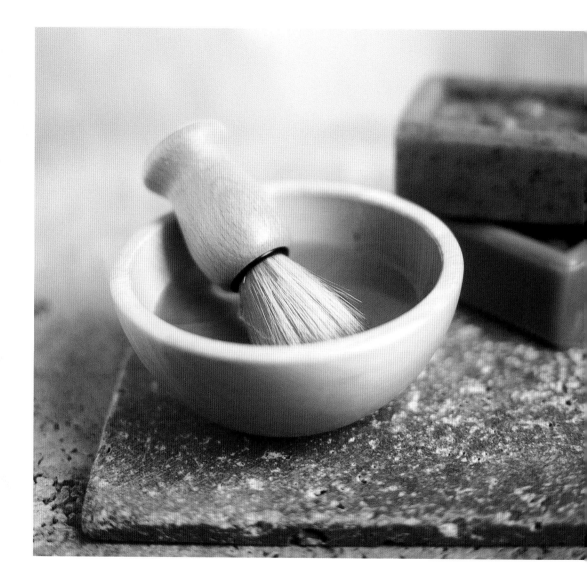

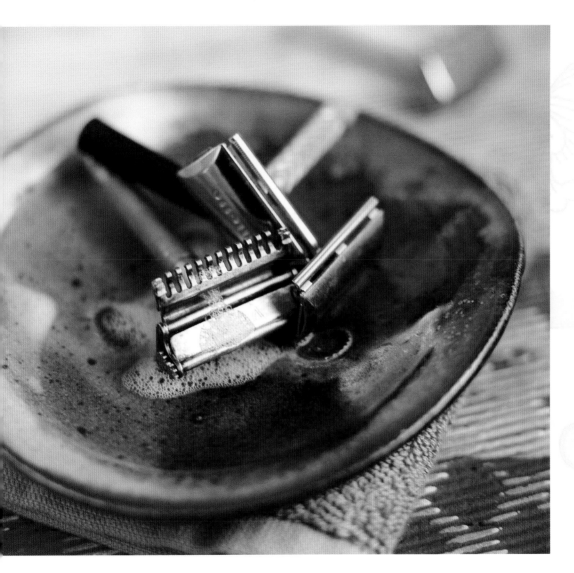

grooming for men

shave oil

normal/dry skin

ingredients

30 ml (1 fl oz) grapeseed oil

20 ml ($1/2$ fl oz) coconut oil

4 drops cedarwood essential oil

6 drops sandalwood essential oil

2 drops lavender essential oil

method

Combine all the ingredients in a dark bottle. Wash your face. Place a warm cloth over your whole face and leave on for 2 minutes. Remove the cloth. Apply the oil mixture then shave. There is no need to wash off the oil residue.

shave rash oil

normal/dry/sensitive skin

ingredients

20 ml ($1/2$ fl oz) evening primrose oil (or borage seed oil)

1 teaspoon calendula-infused oil

10 drops lavender essential oil

10 drops German chamomile essential oil

method

Combine the ingredients. Use a small amount over rash after shaving. Leave on for 5 minutes, then wash off.

anti-irritant shave gel

sensitive skin

A non-sudsy shave gel for irritated and inflamed skin. Horsetail extract is available from health food stores.

ingredients

50 g (1³/4 oz) aloe vera gel

3 teaspoons sweet almond oil

1 capsule horsetail extract

4 drops carrot seed essential oil

2 drops lavender essential oil

2 drops sandalwood essential oil

method

Combine the aloe vera gel, almond oil and horsetail extract (prick the horsetail extract capsule and squeeze out the contents) and mix thoroughly. Add the essential oils and stir through gently. Use when shaving or apply to the skin after shaving.

after-shave balm

all skin types

ingredients

75 g (2^{1}/$_{2}$ oz/1^{1}/$_{2}$ cups) linseeds
150 ml (5 fl oz) boiling water
40 g (1^{1}/$_{2}$ oz) aloe vera gel
2 teaspoons evening primrose oil
1 teaspoon apricot kernel oil
^{1}/$_{2}$ teaspoon vitamin E oil
5 drops sandalwood essential oil
1 drop ylang-ylang essential oil

method

Soak the linseeds in the boiling water overnight or simmer on the stove until a gel forms, strain, then discard the liquid. Add the aloe vera gel, evening primrose oil, apricot kernel oil, vitamin E oil and the essential oils and mix thoroughly. Spoon into a glass container and store in a cool place.

Apply over skin after shaving or after sun exposure.

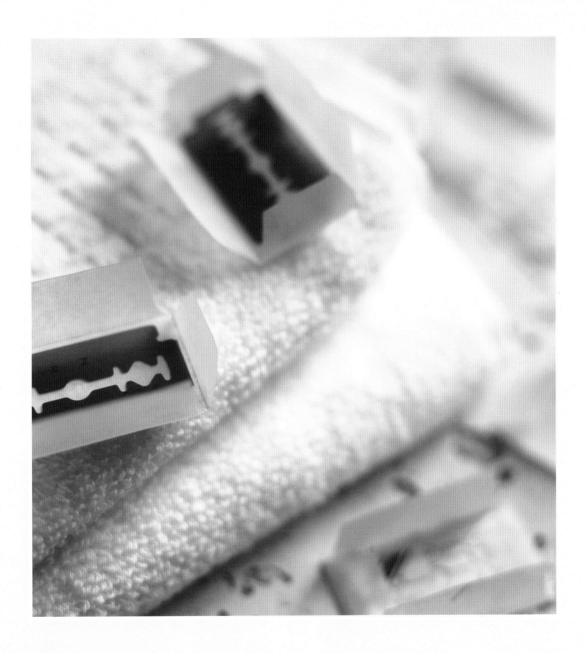

cologne spritzer

all skin types

ingredients

70 ml (2¹/4 fl oz) 100% proof vodka

20 drops orange essential oil

10 drops lemon essential oil

4 drops cedarwood essential oil

6 drops sandalwood essential oil

3 drops ylang-ylang essential oil

30 ml (1 fl oz) distilled water

method

Combine all the ingredients except the distilled water into a dark bottle. Shake well and leave to stand for up to 48 hours. Add the distilled water. Leave for at least 48 hours.

The cologne will be much stronger if you let it stand for 2–3 weeks. To use, spray all over your body, avoiding the face area.

citrus refresh

all skin types

ingredients

55 ml (1^3/$_4$ fl oz) vodka

25 ml (^{3}/$_4$ fl oz) distilled water

25 ml (^{3}/$_4$ fl oz) witch hazel

20 drops orange essential oil

15 drops lime essential oil

5 drops patchouli essential oil

5 drops cedarwood essential oil

20 drops benzoin essential oil

method

Combine all the ingredients in a dark bottle and leave to synergize for 3 days.

To use, spray all over your body, avoiding the face area.

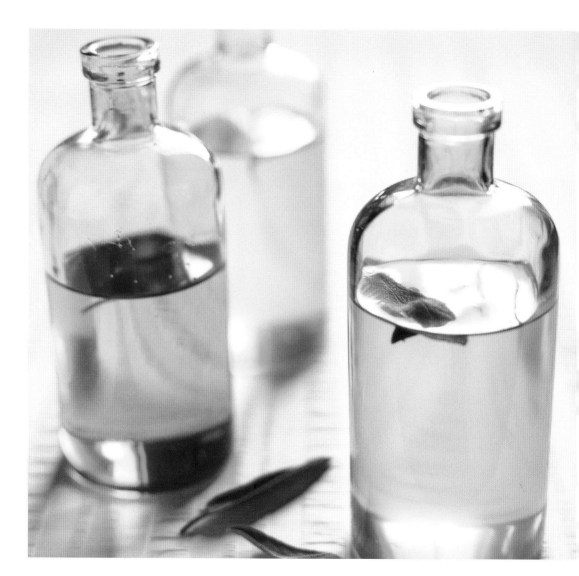

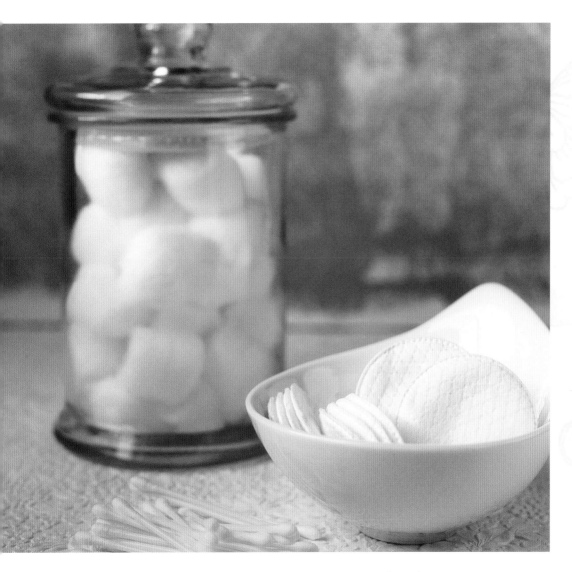

health care

antiseptic balm

all skin types

ingredients

20 g ($^3/_4$ oz) beeswax

20 ml ($^1/_2$ fl oz) calendula-infused oil

30 ml (1 fl oz) apricot kernel oil

20 g ($^3/_4$ oz) aloe vera gel

1 teaspoon St John's Wort

8 drops lavender essential oil

6 drops myrrh essential oil

6 drops frankincense essential oil

method

Melt the beeswax in the top half of a double boiler. Add the calendula-infused and apricot kernel oils. Heat together and leave to cool slightly. Add the aloe vera gel, St John's Wort and the essential oils and mix thoroughly. Spoon into glass containers and store in a cool place. Apply on rashes, bites, stings, fungal infections, acne scars and other scars.

insect bites

all skin types

Slowly add 2 teaspoons demineralized water to 20 g ($^3/_4$ oz) bicarbonate of soda (baking soda) and 20 g ($^3/_4$ oz) kaolin clay and mix thoroughly. Add 3 drops lemon essential oil, 2 drops tea tree essential oil and 4 drops lavender essential oil and stir well.

Apply to *insect bites* only. Can be used for bites from mosquitos, sand flies, fleas, etc.

tea tree after-wax oil

all skin types

This antiseptic, antibacterial oil can help soothe and calm irritated skin and minimize ingrown hairs.

ingredients

30 ml (1 fl oz) sweet almond oil

20 ml ($1/2$ fl oz) apricot kernel oil

10 drops lavender essential oil

5 drops tea tree essential oil

method

Combine all the ingredients and pour into a dark bottle. Shake well. Rub lightly into waxed skin (avoiding the genital area).

mouthwash

ingredients

20 ml ($^1/2$ fl oz) brandy

80 ml ($2^1/2$ fl oz/$^1/3$ cup) aloe vera juice

3 drops peppermint essential oil

1 drop tea tree essential oil

2 drops eucalyptus essential oil

2 drops myrrh essential oil

method

Combine all the ingredients in a glass bottle. Add 1 teaspoon of the mixture to half a glass of water and gargle.

deodorant spray

ingredients

55 ml ($1^3/4$ fl oz) witch hazel (or vodka)

55 ml ($1^3/4$ fl oz) demineralized water

1 teaspoon vegetable glycerine

10 drops patchouli essential oil

10 drops bergamot essential oil

5 drops lemon essential oil

10 drops cypress essential oil

method

Combine all the ingredients in a glass bottle with a spray nozzle. Leave to synergize for 3 days before using.

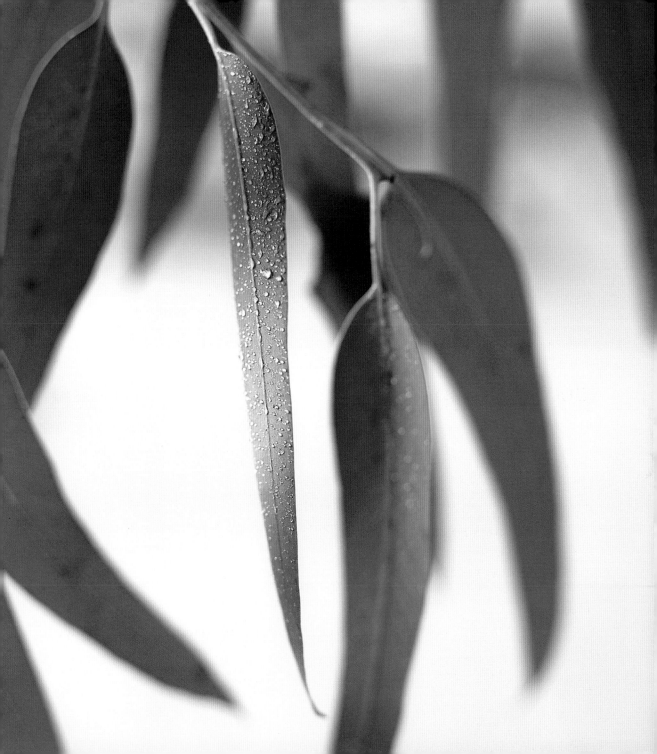

index